ADVANCE PRAISE FOR

The
Practical
Cyclist

Discover or rediscover the simple pleasures and benefits of riding a bike with Chip Haynes as your guide, shaman, coach. It's Andy Rooney meets Jerry Seinfeld meets Ghandi meets your favorite science teacher, all on two wheels. In a clear, unpretentious voice, Chip delivers a wonderful, practical thesis that will forever change — for the better — the way you think about bicycles.

— Jim Joyce, Editor
The Bicycle Book: Wit, Wisdom & Wanderings

This may sound like heresy, but reading Chip Haynes' delightful book, *The Practical Cyclist*, is almost as much fun as riding my bike. Curled up on my sofa, Chip's book in hand, I have yet to be charged by a howling dog or cursed by a motorist consumed by road rage. On the other hand, while reading the book I didn't burn as many calories, and I feel really guilty about wolfing down a pint of ice cream by myself.

— Jeff Klinkenberg
St. Petersburg Times

The
Practical
Cyclist

The
Practical
Cyclist

BICYCLING FOR REAL PEOPLE

Chip Haynes

796.6
Haynes

4/09

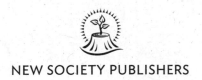

NEW SOCIETY PUBLISHERS

Cataloging in Publication Data:
A catalog record for this publication is available from the National Library of Canada.

Cover design by Diane McIntosh and Chip Haynes.
Illustrations by Chip Haynes.

Printed in Canada.
First printing April 2009

Paperback ISBN: 978-0-86571-633-9

Inquiries regarding requests to reprint all or part of *The Practical Cyclist* should be addressed to New Society Publishers at the address below.

To order directly from the publishers, please call toll-free (North America) 1-800-567-6772, or order online at www.newsociety.com

Any other inquiries can be directed by mail to:

New Society Publishers
P.O. Box 189, Gabriola Island, BC V0R 1X0, Canada
(250) 247-9737

New Society Publishers' mission is to publish books that contribute in fundamental ways to building an ecologically sustainable and just society, and to do so with the least possible impact on the environment, in a manner that models this vision. We are committed to doing this not just through education, but through action. This book is one step toward ending global deforestation and climate change. It is printed on Forest Stewardship Council-certified acid-free paper that is 100% post-consumer recycled (100% old growth forest-free), processed chlorine free, and printed with vegetable-based, low-VOC inks, with covers produced using FSC-certified stock. Additionally, New Society purchases carbon offsets based on an annual audit, operating with a carbon-neutral footprint. For further information, or to browse our full list of books and purchase securely, visit our website at: www.newsociety.com

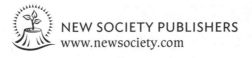
NEW SOCIETY PUBLISHERS
www.newsociety.com

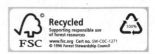
Recycled
Supporting responsible use
of forest resources
FSC
www.fsc.org Cert no. SW-COC-1271
© 1996 Forest Stewardship Council

BOOKS FOR WISER LIVING RECOMMENDED BY MOTHER EARTH NEWS

Today, more than ever before, our society is seeking ways to live more conscientiously. To help bring you the very best inspiration and information about greener, more sustainable lifestyles, *Mother Earth News* is recommending select New Society Publishers' books to its readers. For more than 30 years, *Mother Earth* has been North America's "Original Guide to Living Wisely," creating books and magazines for people with a passion for self-reliance and a desire to live in harmony with nature. Across the countryside and in our cities, New Society Publishers and *Mother Earth* are leading the way to a wiser, more sustainable world.

Dedicated to
The Lovely JoAnn,
of course

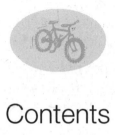

Contents

INTRODUCTIONS ...
Are In Order

A S ODD AS IT MAY SEEM, I'M GOING TO START BY TELLING YOU WHAT this book is not: it's not a bicycle repair manual. (That would explain the total lack of technical illustrations, wouldn't it?) There are plenty of good books out there on that great and ever-expanding subject, and I see no need for me to add to the pile with this book. Nor is this going to be one of those sweaty fitness books claiming to give you abs of steel and buns of cinnamon. You really don't have to be some sort of outstanding physical specimen to ride a bicycle. I'm sure not, and yet I do. (Ride a bicycle, that is.) And that's more in keeping with what this book is all about: the idea that just about anyone — even me and yes, even you — can go out and ride a bicycle, do so safely and comfortably, have a good time, and maybe drive their car just a little bit less. That's really what it's all about.

Well, that and the Hokey-Pokey.

Now before you start to worry over that last crack about driving your car a little bit less, let me tell you this right up front: I have no intention of beating you over the head with an organic, free-range, well-hugged tree to try and make you feel guilty about driving your car and not giving it up for the good of the planet. I drive a truck. There. I've said it. You know the truth. Let's not dwell on it. I won't ask you what you drive, and you won't ask me to help when you want to move. Fair enough? This is a book about the joys of bicycling — and there are many. You don't have to be a skinny road racer, a muscled mountain biker, or a tattooed urban bike messenger to get out there on a regular bicycle, actually going somewhere — and enjoy it. It can be done, and if I do this right, this book will help you do just that: enjoy riding your bicycle. And if you want to get a tattoo, be sure and ask your Mom first.

Don't look for specific brand names in this book. I'm not going to tell you what brand bicycle to buy, or even what brand bike I ride. It honestly doesn't matter *what* we ride, only *that* we ride. In the same vein, it doesn't matter if next year's Fizznodal 24 Speed Extra Special is really any better a bike than last year's Borsnorp 21 Speed with Added Fiber. I don't care, and neither should you. You don't even have to buy a new bike. There are plenty of great used ones out there. Bikes very seldom go bad, and it's difficult to buy a truly bad bicycle these days, new or used. The truth is, any brand name information I might be tempted to put in this book right now would be hopelessly outdated by the time you read it. Models change every year, and even the same model can change from year to year. In

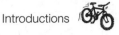

addition, not all bike brands or models are available everywhere in the world — and I have no idea where you are. You
could drop me a line, but by then it would be too late. Models
change. I will tell you what to look for when you buy a bicycle
(wherever you are), something about where to buy your bicycle and why you should buy it there. Hopefully, by the time
you've read this book, you'll be a pretty fair judge of horseflesh
yourself, and the sales staff will all assume
you know what you're doing the moment
you walk in the door. They make that
mistake with me all the time.

   And who am I? I'm just a
guy that likes to ride my bike.
I learned to ride a bike back
when the earth's crust was still
warm and dinosaurs roamed the
earth. It was also called the 1950s. I rode my bicycle — a somewhat larger bicycle, thankfully — all through my teenage school
years which, as you might imagine, made me immensely popular. (*So* not really.) Still, I kept at it and enjoyed, like so many
that lived through it, the Big Bike Boom of the 70s which, for
me, more than made up for the weird big hair and slimy plastic
clothes of that decade. I wisely chose to totally ignore the disco
era, parked my bicycle for a bit — OK, for twenty years — and
then one day, I saw it: a small English folding bike out in front
of the pawn shop downtown. It was for sale. Uh-oh. I was in
trouble. I wanted that bike. I *needed* that bike.

   OK, yes, as a matter of fact, I did still have my bike from the
70s, but this was different: that little bike needed me as much

as I needed it. It needed saving. I agonized about it over the weekend (I had seen it on a Friday), and the following Monday I bought the bike and brought it home. I had a new friend. I took a bit of time to go over it and make sure it was in good running order (it was), and it fit me better than a glove. (It's surprisingly difficult to pedal a glove anywhere with any success whatsoever.) That was in late November, and by the first Monday in January, I took the plunge: I rode that little three-speed folding bike to work for the first time. Many more times followed. Many years' worth of many times. That is one fun bike. That was back in 1997, and I'm still riding that bike now. (Well, not *right* now. Right now I'm sitting at a desk.) I put ten miles on my little folding bike yesterday and I'll put another six on it today. It still fits. And somewhere along the way, I began to write about bicycling, which brings us mercifully closer to the end of this introduction.

I know how annoyed I get when I read endless thank-yous in other people's books. (So why do I read them?) As a result, I plan to keep this part quite short: three people get thanked here. That's it. Just three. You can skip over this bit if you want, but I still have to say it:

The first thank-you goes out to my wonderful wife, the lovely JoAnn. She puts up with my wacky interest in bicycles and tolerates those seemingly endless trips to the bicycle shop for little widgets and doohickies. She's very understanding, and I love her more than life itself. More than bicycles, even. This book is dedicated to her, as am I.

My second thank-you goes out to Mason St. Clair of Nashville, Tennessee. Mason is the editor and publisher of the

Wire Donkey, a hardcopy-only bicycle newsletter that he mails out once a month to a handful of the faithful. I started writing articles for Mason's *Wire Donkey* many years ago, and still to this day send in one or two each week. To date, I've sent him over 1200 articles on bicycling, and he's put every last one of them in his great little newsletter. I have to thank him for giving me that start in this sort of thing, and putting up with my many typos. Thnaks, Mason.

OK, the last person I really have to thank: Ingrid Witvoet at New Society Publishers. Through an odd and random crossing of paths, we met (cyberspacially speaking) and she was willing to entertain my proposal to write this book. She *trusted* me to write this book. I figured she had some sort of proposal quota to fill, but hey, I'll play along. If you're reading this, it means that the kind folks at New Society Publishers are truly understanding people indeed and have indulged me in this endeavor. Here's hoping this works out. Thank you, Ingrid.

If you have a complaint about this book, call New Society Publishers. If you have a compliment about this book, call New Society Publishers. If you just want to go for a bicycle ride — call me. I'm ready!

Now read on.

WHY BOTHER? —
You Know You Want To

L ET ME GIVE YOU THE GOOD NEWS FIRST (SINCE THERE REALLY IS NO
bad news): riding a bicycle is fun. It's that simple. That's
why I do it, and that's why you should, too. Sure, there are
other reasons to ride a bike, and we'll get to those in a minute,
but you need to know that riding a bicycle is more fun than
driving a car — even on rainy days. As a matter of fact, I hate
getting wet, but don't mind riding my bicycle in the rain (properly attired for the weather, of course). I can't explain it, but
there it is: even the rain is more fun on a bike. And those warm,
sunny days are beyond compare when you are on your bicycle.

There's just something inherently more pleasant about being
out in the world on a bicycle, versus being stuck inside a car,
watching the world go sailing by the tinted windows. Even with
the windows rolled down, it's just not the same. The joy of cycling

must have something to do with being out there under your own power, the feeling of being so much more in control of all that is going on around you, and all of that unfiltered fresh air. It gets to you. Sure, you drive the car, but you *power* the bike. You are both engine and engineer. It's all you, and it feels great.

So many of us learned to ride a bike as a child, and did ride a bike right up to the day we got our driver's license. After that, the bike was cast aside, and it was all about speed and power and four wheels and dual exhausts and, well, somewhere along the line we lost track of something there. Sure, the car is faster and takes less physical effort, but there's still something missing in the experience when you drive. The drive might be exhilarating, but the car is not all that satisfying. More often than not, we're stuck in traffic and, harkening back to the days of the horse, it doesn't smell all that good. Especially if you get a lot of them in one place. (Cars or horses, either one.) We all see the car commercials that show empty roads and wide open vistas, but the reality of the world is quite different. The car, once a symbol of freedom of movement, is now a static display on a road clogged with millions of other cars, all wanting to go, go, go — but all stuck in traffic and going nowhere fast, their drivers stuck behind the wheel of a machine that cannot move because *everyone* wants to move. I see this every day — as I pedal by them on my bicycle. It's sad, really. If only they had ridden a bicycle instead. Maybe next time they'll ride a bike. Maybe?

Bicycling For Your Health? Good Idea!

Aside from actually being able to get somewhere when the city is gridlocked with bumper-to-bumper traffic, there are other great reasons for riding a bicycle instead of driving a car. Your personal health is a really good reason — maybe the best reason of all. Bicycling is a wonderful low-impact form of exercise. It's easy on the legs and knees (much easier than walking or running), and you really don't have to go at it like a crazy (sweaty) person to get the benefits of a good workout on a bike. Even a modest pace on a bicycle should be good for burning about 400 calories an hour, and it takes very little to boost that pace and burn even more. You can do this — at your own speed.

You've heard the old adage about weight loss being all about diet and exercise, but here's the truth: if all you did was ride your bicycle all day, even at an easy pace, you probably wouldn't have to worry about what you ate — only that you ate *enough*. Sounds like fun, doesn't it? Of course, we all can't just drop what we're doing and go ride our bikes from sun up to sun down. But many of us can ride just a little every day, and every little bit helps. My normal day sees me riding for at least 40 minutes, 20 in the morning and another 20 in the late afternoon. No, it's not an epic ride either way, but it's enough to help — and it makes me feel good. On my days off, I ride a little more, and it feels even better.

Riding a bicycle, even a little bit, helps work your heart and lungs and keeps your legs limber and your muscles in shape. You even get an upper-body workout with the steering and balance. You're constantly turning your head to see what's going on around you, working your neck muscles, and the brain is going full blast trying to process all of that information and take it all in. Congratulations — you're multi-tasking just by riding a bike! Yes, you can ride a bike without breaking a sweat if you want to. I do that all the time. No need to work too hard at it. The whole idea is to have fun and maybe get somewhere in the process. Even around the block is a whole new experience compared to driving in the car. From the seat of your bicycle, the neighborhood you thought you knew (by car) becomes an entirely new adventure on two wheels in the wide open great outdoors. You're going to see so many things you never saw before, you'll wonder how you missed so much of it. (And why you waited so long.)

In addition to the considerable physical benefits of cycling, there's a wonderful mental side to it as well. This goes beyond the mundane mental exercise of watching for traffic and balancing the bike as you pedal along and wonder if that dog over there is on a leash or if we are about to go for a race. Bicycling instills the rider with a sense of great anticipation on every ride. Where will you go next? What will you see there? And does that rear tire look soft to you? It's a never-ending parade. There's always more to take in and another place to go. (But be sure and check those tires before you go. Especially that back one.)

In the original bike boom in the 1890s, the bicycle was seen as the most welcome replacement for the horse, in that the bike required very little care, both in use and in storage. When not in use, it could be parked in the hall for weeks at a time and totally ignored. Try that with a horse — any horse. Even a small horse. And let me know how that works out, will you? Of course, the original advantage of the bicycle over the horse was much more daring, if not actually scandalous, in those staid and proper Victorian times: the bicycle could convey a man or a

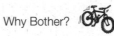

woman (or a man *and* a woman) from the crowded urban city to the rural, empty countryside without the need for anyone to know. No need to rent a horse and carriage, no need to deal with stable hands or the men at the local livery. Just wheel your bicycle out and go. *No chaperone.* It was positively unheard of. What was the world coming to? Oh, my!

That same thrill of being ever so slightly scandalous can still be had today, just by riding off on your bike. Take off across town on your bicycle, and no one needs to know where you are. Few people will see you, and fewer still will recognize you. Most of them aren't looking for *you* anyway — they're looking for your *car*. (How many times have we all heard, "Didn't I see you parked at ..."? No, that was my truck. I was inside.) Fool them. Be invisible. Ride a bike — it feels good to be adventurous. In this day and age of instant and constant connectivity, the idea of traveling totally detached and out of touch with the rest of the technical, modern world most certainly does have its appeal. No phones to answer, no messages coming in, nothing to reply to. You are your own person, if only for an hour or so as you ride your bike. You can go where you like, when you like, and change what you like in a heartbeat — and then change your plans again. The bicycle offers you a freedom the car could never equal: the freedom of traveling virtually unseen by the rest of the world. Use the power wisely, my young apprentice. (But have fun!)

The other side of that power of invisibility is the sense of empowerment it gives you to be able to go somewhere on your bike. Remember the feeling you had as a kid, the first time you rode your bicycle out of sight of your house? That feeling is still out there, waiting for you. And it still feels *good*. That feeling of accomplishment and wild adventure can be a real boost, even if all you do is pedal over to the local store you've been to (by car) a thousand times. You did it! All by yourself! On your bike! Ha! Take *that*, world! OK, OK, let's not get carried away here. Not yet, anyway.

Still, if you ride your bike on a regular basis, you do tend to get an elevated sense of self-worth that could never come from driving a car to the very same places. To drive to work is drudgery. To ride a bike to work is adventure! (Even if you still do just end up at work.) Whoever said it was all about the journey and not the destination was probably riding a bicycle. Maybe it has something to do with the benefits of the exercise involved, or the mental rush of being out there in the wind and sun, with everything all around you, without the car to protect you, but a bicycle ride across town does more for your ego than driving your car across town ever could. No matter what car you drive.

So it comes to this: if you want to feel good, and feel good about yourself, go ride a bike. You don't have to go fast or go far, but you do have to go. Get out there in the wind and the sun (or under the moon!) and see the world around you as you haven't seen it since you were a kid. It's still out there, waiting for you to come back. All you need is a bicycle and a little practice, and the world will be your oyster. *Your oyster?* I never did

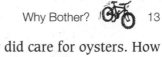

understand that phrase. And I never did care for oysters. How about this: the world will be your happy beagle. Doesn't that sound like a lot more fun?

In It For The Money? That Works, Too

We've talked about health, now let's talk about wealth. Here's a screamingly obvious fact of life: riding a bicycle is less expensive than driving a car. *It's not free*, but it is cheaper. That last statement is really important, and yet often overlooked by people who are looking into bicycling, but then go into sticker shock when they see what a good bicycle can cost. Or a great bicycle, for that matter. Yes, if you want to, you *can* pay as much for a bicycle as you would for a car. (I'm not joking here. You really could. Honest.) The difference is, a bicycle that expensive would be absolutely top-of-the-line, a hand-made work of art — and the car would be just a car. If a thing of beauty is a joy forever, as Mr. Keats says it is, then a fine bicycle is all that and more. Did Keats ride a bicycle? If he did in 1818, when he wrote "Endymion" (and the above line about eternal beauty and joy), then he must have been among the first in the world to do so, and would be astounded by the beautiful bicycles we ride today. Bicycles, in this regard, are much like everything else in life: you get what you pay for.

I have a bicycle I bought over thirty years ago. I paid a tidy sum for it. I paid a tidy sum for it by *today's* standards. It is, in the words of Keats, a joy forever. And I know that because for what I paid for that bike, I get a lot of joy: all I have to do is pump up the tires and that bike is ready for an epic ride right now — thirty years later. It has not aged. It has not suffered. Try that with a thirty-year-old car. Of course, I also have bicycles I have paid *nothing* for, and they're nice, too. The thing is, you get more for your money with a bicycle than you will ever get with a car. The quality is there at a much lower price point. Often for free.

But how much will you save if you ride a bike? That's what you want to know, isn't it? First off, you have to understand that most of the expense of owning a car doesn't come from driving it. It comes from simply owning it. That means it can just sit there, doing nothing and going nowhere, and it will still cost you money. (How's *that* for annoying?) The car payments, the insurance, the depreciation — the entropy — they all go right on, day after day, year after year, whether you drive the thing or not. By not driving, you save a little on gas, a little on oil, and maybe some wear and tear on the tires (that are aging anyway as we speak). Oh, and your battery's going flat, too, you know. If you want to ride a bike to save money on your car, you're going to have to sell your car — and let's not get hasty here. It's OK if you ride your bike and keep your car. You will save a little. Just not a lot. You need to know that.

I once figured out that my truck was costing me one thousandth of its purchase price every day, seven days a week, 365 days a year. That really adds up. I still have the truck, but mostly, I ride my bike and still save a bundle of money. Here's how: since I ride my bicycle to work, my wife can use our truck to go shopping and run errands. Since we don't need to buy a second vehicle for me to go to work (it's only three miles/five kilometers between my home and the office), she doesn't have to get a job to pay for the second car we don't need. So she stays

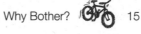

home, I pedal to work, and life is good. Yes, the bicycle really can save you a bundle of money if you do it right.

The other place where the bicycle can save you money goes back to the bicycle helping to keep you healthy. Healthy people spend less time and money being sick. Sounds stupid when I put it that way, doesn't it? Let me try this again: by using bicycling to maintain your health and fitness, you need not spend money on a health club you won't use, a neglected home exercise machine that will just take up space, and any number of medications and medical services you might need if you didn't get out there and pedal that bike just a little. Keeping yourself healthy, keeping the weight off, and moving around on a bicycle is by far the best prescription for good health and long life that you can have. And it's certainly among the cheapest. More money saved right there. Maybe a lot more. You're welcome.

So what does it cost to own a bicycle? It would be foolish for me to quote a price that would make no sense to you by the time you read it here, so let me put it like this: if I spend one-tenth of what I make in one week on my bicycles for required maintenance in one year, that's a lot. That's just to replace worn-out tires and tubes, buy tube repair kits and replace the odd broken cable. And that would be a very busy year for me for bicycle maintenance. Now yes, it's true that I really do spend a lot more than that on my bicycles, but it's almost all voluntary. Once you buy the bike and get it set up the way you want it, the day-to-day expenses are below minimal — they are virtually non-existent. It's very easy to go for long stretches of time — for months — and not spend anything at all on your bicycle. But when the time comes, you need to know that you will have to. Things do wear out. Tires, tubes, cables, chains, they will all need to be replaced in time. Even seats give out eventually. (Mine and the bike's.) Every time I have to spend some money on my bike, I think about how much I'm saving not having to maintain a second car. That makes me smile — and I usually end up spending more on my bike.

Saving The Planet — One Bike At A Time

One big angle for many bicycle riders is the environmental advantage of riding a bike instead of driving a car. You don't have to be a hard-core green earth activist to see that riding a bicycle is a good idea from an earth-loving global point of view. Even if you only ride a little, that means you're driving a little less. And that's good. Sure, in the big scheme of things your not driving your car today probably won't tip the scales toward green to any great (or even noticeable) degree, but *you* know you're doing it, and that does count for something. Seven billion people on planet earth, and you rode your bike today. Go team.

Seriously, it does matter, and it may help more than you think (and certainly more than I'm letting on). If you ride your bike, people will *see* you riding your bike — and then maybe they'll ride *their* bike. It could happen. You could start a trend. Be a movement. Lead the parade. All on your bike. While Lao Tzu always went on about a long journey starting with a single step, any great movement starts with a single person. In your town, that one person could be you. You could make a difference — all by riding your bike. Then again, you might ride alone for years and never know if you've done any good at all. Life's funny that way. I'm laughing on the inside.

One thing I have noticed is this: as I have ridden my bike over the years, I have become more aware of how I live the rest of my life, and often choose to do better than I did, greenly speaking. I would never portray myself as some great environmental guru, but a good friend of mine did recently label me a "green freak." To my face, no less. I'm not sure it was meant as a compliment, but I took it as one. *Cool.* I *can* be taught! And I am doing better. I do try to make better choices. I recycle, I bring my own bags to the store and yes, many times, I ride to the store on my bicycle. Around here where I live, that must be all you have to do to earn the title of "green freak." Our standards are noticeably lower here, it would seem. So do keep that in mind: if you ride a bicycle, you run the risk of developing a certain *reputation*. Not to mention a whole new (greener) outlook on life. It's just a chance you'll have to take. It's OK. It's worth it.

As a cyclist, your view of the environment — or what's left of it — is going to be considerably enhanced — make that tainted — by all that you will see around you as you ride. The real world outside is not always green and lovely and pristine. The hand of man is not always kind. That's the polite, poetic way of saying there's a lot of trash out there along the road, and we put it all there ourselves, one stupid piece at a time. If that doesn't make an environmentalist out of you, nothing will. Of course, getting out on the road on your bicycle also gives you the chance to do something about that. I've picked up some pretty cool stuff out there over the years that other people have thrown out. Whole bicycles even. One man's trash, and all that. Go team, indeed.

I have to warn you: once you've been riding your bicycle for a while, even just around your own neighborhood, your friends and neighbors, your coworkers and relatives, will all look at you differently. Sometimes they'll squint. You are no longer the person they thought they knew. Now you are a *bicyclist* — and that, to many people who are not, is a whole different sort of animal. Your reputation will change. I'd like to say it will be for the better, but hey, it's your reputation and none of my business. But everyone who knows you will think differently of you, and people who don't know you will make stuff up. You will be The Cyclist. Can you handle that? It will be a new image for you. You'll be your own action figure. It could be a good thing, but many people look at a bicyclist — even a practical one — as something less than normal, instead of something more.

H. G. Wells once famously said that he did not despair for the future of the human race when he saw an adult on a bicycle. That's great, Herbie, but out here in the modern (car-driven) world, an adult on a bicycle is more often cause for concern and question, and that question would have to be: "Why aren't you driving a car?" The trick here is to look like you mean it. If you're going to ride your bicycle (and you are), then by all means *ride* your bicycle. Sit right up, back straight (good posture!), hold your head up high and give everyone you meet a big smile and a friendly wave. Hey, blow them a kiss if you like. Really confuse them. Too many people ride bicycles like it was the result of some unpleasant court order. Don't be a grouch about it. This is fun, and that fun should show through when you ride. If riding a bicycle isn't more fun than driving a car, there's something wrong and we need to fix it. Maybe the tires are low. Have you checked the brakes? Is the seat too low? Check the tires first. Make the bike ride all the fun it should be, and it will show. People will envy you. No, really. They will. They may not actually say that they do, but they do. They told me so.

That Edgy Counter-Culture Thing

The other angle, when it comes to your image on a bicycle, is to jump right in with both feet and really embrace that cool, edgy, counter-culture side of bicycling. It *is* different. In far too many modern societies, it is not yet a common, everyday thing to see an adult on a bicycle. (In Wells' day, yes, but now, sadly, not so much.) For a large part of the modern mechanized world, to ride a bike is a very different thing. It stands out. *You* stand out when you're on a bike. In a very small way, if you only ride a bike and not own a car, you have denied the government a certain amount of taxation and regulation. Not enough to get on anyone's naughty list, mind you, but enough to maybe save yourself a little pocket change — and make you look larger than life to those who drive. Since I have my feet in both worlds, my reputation on either side of that fence is nothing special. I drive, but I also ride. (Or do I ride, but also drive? I suspect the latter.) It's either the best of times or the worst of times, and I'm never sure which. Still, there's no denying the counter-culture aspect of bicycling, and for many that angle does have a certain draw and charm. Be the Cyclist. Even when they aren't looking.

You can take that bicycle of yours and build a whole new image — a whole new life — around those two wheels. You can be the secret rebel you always wanted to be — the one you promised yourself you *would* be, way back when. Traveling by bike you're under the radar and off the map. Nobody's fool (but your own). Go ahead, live life on the edge. Ride a bicycle like you really mean it. Give the hat a bit of a tilt. Wear two kinds of plaid. Just remember what I said about asking your Mom before you get that tattoo.

A BRIEF HISTORY OF BIKE —
Sorry, Dr. Hawking

M Y FIRST BIKE WAS A TINY ONE-SPEED WITH SOLID RUBBER TIRES, and I managed to break that bicycle in half riding up over a curb. My instant ownership of two small unicycles was remedied by a quick bit of welding (Thanks, Dad!), and my bicycling has continued — with some interruptions — to this day. At least none of my other bikes have broken in half. (I've gotten much smoother at that curb-jumping thing.)

Bicycles themselves began as welcome replacements for the horse some two hundred years ago. Very welcome replacements, indeed. The first "hobby horses" had no pedals, gears, driving mechanisms, or even steering. And they weren't, judging from the drawings, very comfortable to ride, either. But they smelled better than horses and ate less, and that was all it took. The Comte de Sivrac demonstrated what may well have been the very first ancestor to today's bicycles in the Royal Palace Gardens of Paris in 1791. Two wheels attached to a padded cross beam with rigid (non-steering) forks. The model of simplicity, if not outright pain. But was it the first? Maybe not. The same sort of machine can be found in a stained glass window in the church of Stoke Poges near Windsor in England, dating back to 1642. So the first cyclists were cherubs? So it would seem. We cyclists were in good company right from the start.

It wasn't until 1817 that Baron Drais von Sauerbronn, in Mannheim, Germany, figured out how to steer the thing by passing the front wheel's mounting fork through the cross frame and adding a lever at the top: A-ha! Handlebars! The very thing we still have today, more or less. The hobby horse, or dandy horse, was now the Draisienne. And bicycling took a giant leap forward, one step at a time.

It's a wonder this thing caught on at all. It wasn't all that light or easy to push these early "bicycles", and they weren't really comfortable for sitting *or* riding. So, then: why *did* the bicycle, even in this crude form, become so popular? Simple: it was cool, or at least the early 19th century equivalent of cool. Quite the boulevard cruiser, in those distant days long before tail fins, big engines and even AM radio. (Remember *AM radio?*) Dandies plied the avenues, all over-dressed and under-equipped to deal with their new-found life on the road. But they were *cool*, and that's all that mattered — even way back then. The bicycle was not originally intended as a form of transportation or even sport. Like so many other (if not all) of men's inventions, its original purpose and intent was simple: to impress the ladies. Some things never change. Men don't. But it must have worked: we're still here, and so are the bicycles. And we men are still trying to impress the ladies. Sometimes with our bicycle.

While the first velocipedes featured equal-sized wheels but no way to drive them, the first common mechanical propulsion systems were nearly the machine's undoing. There was none to begin with, except for the rider pushing it along with his feet to the ground on either side of the most uncomfortable horizontal beam. It was only a matter of time before someone figured out that a set of treadles connected to the rear wheel could be used to drive the machine forward, with the advantage of getting the rider's feet up off the ground and out of the muck and mire. (Horses were very popular back then, remember. That muck and mire smelled bad and worse.) The year was about 1840, and the man was Scotsman Kirkpatrick Macmillan. Of course, no one thought this treadle-driven thing of his would work. It was obvious, even to the village idiot, that if you picked up *both* your feet, the thing would fall over, right? After a few well-attended public demonstrations of balance, skill and propulsion, the idea became a bit more accepted, bureaucrats and village idiots excepted.

So treadle propulsion caught on, but inventors kept inventing. (The bicycle, by the way, is one of the most "invented" things on earth. People are always trying something new with it, even today.) Right about 1861, Pierre Michaux figured out how to put a crank and pedals on the now steerable front wheel, and his son Ernest built the beast. Not only did it work, but given the way they lived in Paris, just about everyone in town saw that it worked. The resulting aptly-named "boneshaker" still featured iron-shod rims on wood spoke wheels and a very solid frame, hence the nickname. But it worked well, and offered a simpler drive system than that Scottish treadle thing. It was Paris, and it was popular, and life was good. Up to a point, anyway.

The point was that those small wheels meant small speeds with that direct drive system, so it wasn't long before the front drive wheel got bigger to make it go faster. And then it got bigger and bigger and — well, you get the scary picture: the penny-farthing, or high-wheeler, was born. Just eight years after the Michaux boneshaker, which offered a 36" front wheel, one Charles Spencer in England was already touting the virtues of a 48" front wheel. Spectacular, yes — but safe? Not on your life, which more than a few luckless early riders sacrificed for the pleasure. With four- and five-foot-diameter front wheels quickly being the norm, and seven-foot-diameter monsters not unheard of, the high-wheeler was, under perfect conditions, a graceful sight in motion. (This type of machine, with the large front wheel and small rear wheel, became common enough that these bicycles were called an "Ordinary;" and still are today, by many.) Conditions on the roads of the day, however, were far from perfect or ordinary. All it took was a slight rut, hole, stick, or rock to tip over that ever-so-graceful tall machine. The rider, sitting nearly directly above the front wheel, was at constant risk, and falling from that great height was no laughing matter. It still isn't. Trust me on that one — voice of experience here, with the scars to back it up. In spite of the dangers inherent in the design, Thomas Stevens was the first person to ride a bicycle — a 50" Ordinary — around the world from 1884 to 1887. He was very brave.

It was with good reason that the first of what appear to us now to be normal, everyday bicycles were called "safety" bikes. It was *much* safer to fall from a mere standing height off of those new safety bikes than it was to fall from eight or ten feet up off of an old high-wheeler. You know, these things might just catch on! In truth, with the introduction of the safety bike around 1885, those dangerous high-wheelers disappeared from the cycling scene with astonishing speed. Now the horse had truly met its match, and bicycles of any design were certainly easier to own than a horse, what with the expense of both purchase and maintenance. The earliest known drawings for what we'd call a standard bicycle design were done in 1869 by English mechanic F. W. Shearing. The first to actually build one (in 1876) was George Shergold, also an Englishman. These designs were the first to display nearly equal-sized smaller wheels, a steerable front fork and wheel and a pedal-driven chain drive to the rear wheel — pretty much everything we think of in a normal, everyday bicycle, even today. From there on out, it was all in the details. Many, many details.

Doctor John Boyd Dunlop, a Scottish veterinarian living in Belfast, heard the pleas of his son pedaling on solid tires (or tyres, as the case may be) and invented the first inflatable pneumatic bicycle tires in 1898. Hard to spell, but easy to ride. Thanks, Doctor D. — good job there. All the other bits and pieces got better as well after a hundred years of progress: drive chains got smaller, lighter and stronger. The gear drive systems, whether internal hubs or external changers, did the same. The English Sturmey-Archer company patented the three-speed internal hub in 1902, while Italian Tullio Campagnolo patented the first derailleur in 1940. Legend has it that Frank W. Schwinn penned the original sketch for his company's famous cantilever frame bikes on a napkin in the employee cafeteria in the 1930s. And somewhere along the line, a truly Great Person came up with the finest invention in all of bicycling: asphalt. The planet got paved, and the roads got smooth, and the good life of a practical cyclist just kept getting better.

The wire-spoke wheel became the norm, as did the traditional men's diamond frame design. Wheel sizes still vary a bit. OK, they vary a lot. They always did. But the bikes of a hundred years ago don't look that out of place today. Some of them, anyway. The current trend is to borrow technology from motorcycling, and it's only fair. Motorcycles started out simply as bicycles with — hold on to your hats here — motors bolted on them. What goes around comes around. Now we're seeing the tide turn, and bicycles are showing up in the dealers' showrooms with light-weight motorcycle-type front and rear suspensions, front forks and fork crowns with triple clamps, hydraulically actuated disk brakes front and rear as well as suspended seat posts and handlebar stems. I guess that's better than just mimicking the high handlebars and banana seat, like we used to do. Frames have gone from steel to aluminum to titanium to graphite and carbon fiber. It just keeps getting better, doesn't it? I wonder what we'll see next? At some point, bicycles will fly. No, wait — they already have.

The thing is, in spite of all the invention and innovation over the last hundred years or so, the bicycle is still the bicycle, and a standard, basic one-speed bike is still a joy to own and ride. It's faster than walking, easier than running, and still, a century later, smells better than the horse. No need to bow to contemporary fashion, the bicycle of yesterday is still a good ride today, and the basic bike, unchanged after so many decades, is still a quick and comfortable way to get around.

Eclipsed by the car and often replaced by the motorcycle, the bicycle has managed to hang on and occasionally even prosper. It seems like bicycling becomes a popular fad about every twenty years or so: the post-WWII prosperity boom of the 1950s, the gas crunch/ten-speed thing in the 1970s, and the "mountain bike craze" of the 1990s. (No mountain required, obviously.) So what's it going to be next? You'd better get ready to ride. I predict that better bicycling days are coming again!

THE BICYCLE —
Your Bicycle

I HAVE, OVER THE YEARS, DEVELOPED A SORT OF REPUTATION AS "THE neighborhood bike guy." I ride bikes and I fuss with bikes, both my own and my neighbors'. (Sometimes complete strangers' bikes.) People drop off bikes for me to fix up and give away. I'm the bike guy. And being the bike guy that I am, I tend to get my fair share of bicycle questions from friends, neighbors, coworkers — even from total strangers. (Go figure.) My favorite question is, by far, "Which bike should I buy?" I like that question because it's the easiest to answer: buy the bike that makes you *want* to ride. It's that simple. Nothing else matters. Much like life itself, it's all about passion and desire. Are we still talking bikes here? You bet. Buy the bike that steams your goggles.

Buy the bicycle that makes you want to call in sick to work and go for an all-day bike ride in the opposite direction. Buy the bike that demands that you skip the night class and go out and ride under the full moon. Buy the bike that makes the lawn wait another day to be mowed. Buy the bike that makes your car dusty just sitting in the garage. *That's* the right bike for you. If you don't look at your bicycle and think, "I want to go for a bike ride right now!", you do not have the right bike. And you need the right bike. Don't you?

Let's Go Bike Shopping!

Before I chatter on (and on) about this bike and that bike, maybe I need to say something first about *where* you should buy a bicycle before I talk about *which* bike you should buy. You've got a lot of options on where you buy your bike, and some sources are better than others. None are truly bad, mind you, it's just that there are, well, things to consider about where you buy *before* you buy.

The Number One, Must-See, First Place to buy a bike is your local bicycle shop. I know that sounds obvious, but many people would never think to look there. Why? Because there's a certain mystique about a bicycle shop that can be intimidating to new cyclists looking for their first bike, or someone who is looking to get back into cycling after many years of driving. It's OK. They understand. They'll be gentle. (And if they don't understand and they aren't gentle, we'll just go somewhere else, won't we?) So start with your local bike shop. You'll be glad you did.

Do I need to warn you about sticker shock? Maybe so. Bicycles cost money. That's a hard fact of life, but you're a big kid now, so you can take it. The more you pay for a bike, the

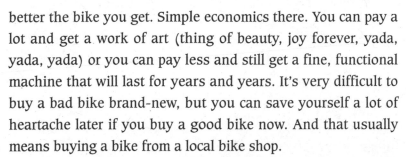

better the bike you get. Simple economics there. You can pay a lot and get a work of art (thing of beauty, joy forever, yada, yada, yada) or you can pay less and still get a fine, functional machine that will last for years and years. It's very difficult to buy a bad bike brand-new, but you can save yourself a lot of heartache later if you buy a good bike now. And that usually means buying a bike from a local bike shop.

Most bike shops carry several different brands of bikes and offer a wide range of models within each brand. That means you can go to one good bike shop and see literally dozens of different bikes that would all work for you. The staff at your local bike shop usually rides bikes themselves (if they don't, you are *so* in the wrong shop) and can offer you some great tips on which models will work for you, and how to set the bike up so it fits and rides just right. Don't like the seat? They can change it. Don't care for the hand grips? They are out of here! Want streamers and a horn? They can make that happen right now. Bike shops not only sell the bike — they make the bike uniquely yours and are there for you in the years ahead whenever you need something for your bike. That service and support is well worth the price. Yes, you probably *will* pay more for a bike at a bike shop, but you are getting so much more bike (and experience) for your money, it's worth it if you plan to keep the bike for more than a month. And you do plan to keep the bike, don't you? I hope so. See you at the bike shop.

I find it a shocking fact of bicycle life that most people do not, in fact, buy their bike at a bike shop. Who knew? Well, OK, I knew. And now you do, too. More bikes are sold, day in and day out, at large (usually discount) department stores. Why is that? Because most folks are more interested in getting "a real deal" than they are in getting a better bike. I call them seasonal bikes, as they usually only last one season — if you're lucky. Department stores do not sell the same bikes you find at a bike shop. Not at that price. The cheaper bikes you find in the toy aisle are made to be sold at a very low price, and the manufacturers get there by using cheaper materials and turning a blind eye to the fit and finish.

No matter where they are sold, bicycles show up at the store (any store) partially assembled (or are they partially disassembled?) in a big brown box. It's up to the store to finish putting the bike together and get it adjusted before it is sold to the customer. In a bicycle shop, those chores are handled by qualified bicycle mechanics who take pride in their work, and want to see that bike do well when it leaves the shop. In a department store, the bike is put together by the first person the manager sees that morning, and if they ever see that bike again, they won't recognize it. The bicycle is not a complex thing, but it does require some intelligence, knowledge, skill and talent to assemble correctly and adjust so that it works as it should. You don't buy a car from a department store — why would you buy a bicycle there?

Yes, the department store bike is cheaper than the bike shop bike. Sometimes *much* cheaper. It can be difficult to ignore the awesome low price, flashing blue lights and mind-numbing background music. Try. Please. If it's all just too much, and you simply must buy your bike at a department store, tell yourself you will sell it or give it away the moment something goes wrong on the bike. Think of it as a "learner bike," a test bike. If you buy a cheap bike at the department store, ride it until you find your One True Bike. (Preferably at a real bicycle shop.) Used as a test bike or learner bike, a department store bike may give you months of good service and let you get a feel for bicycling again. Then again, the wheel could fall off next week. You get what you pay for. I'm just saying.

I have to say this: I once walked into my local grocery store — *the grocery store* — and saw a row of shiny brand-new bicycles for sale up on top of the freezers in the frozen food section. I was amazed, not only at the idea of buying a bicycle at the grocery store, but that they took the time, trouble and effort to hoist each one of those heavy boat anchor bikes all the way up onto those tall freezers. How was I supposed to get one down? How would it fit in my cart? Paper or plastic? Such are the mysteries of life. Those bikes remained there for quite some time, as I recall. As well they should.

The other big source for new bikes is the new source for everything: the Internet. You can just sit right there, in the comfort of your own home, buy a bike, any bike, and have it shipped right to your house and there you are — with a big brown box of bike on your door step. Now what? Unless you feel qualified to put that bike together yourself and adjust it out so it works, you might find yourself in a bit of a spot. (Unless you live near me, of course.) I have put together Internet bikes for friends. It's hilarious. A real grab bag of "What's this?" My favorite was the one that had a crumpled rear fender, in spite of the fact that the whole bike was carefully double-boxed for shipping. How did the fender get so crumpled? The big machine that stapled those two boxes closed did its very best to staple the inside box to the bike itself. Whoopsie! I had to pull the fender off the bike, tap out the dent, sand it down and repaint it. Yeah, that's so much better than buying a bike at a bike shop. Internet shopping might best be described with the old saying "You get what you get, and don't pitch a fit." And good luck getting it put together, by the way. Such a deal.

I'm the kind of guy that tends to blurt out the truth without thinking. Someone asks me what I think, and I'm just dumb enough to tell them. It gets me in trouble every time, but here I go again. The honest truth: your local bike shop does not want to assemble the bike you bought on the Internet. Even if it's a brand they carry. *Especially* if it's a brand they carry. I know it might seem like a good idea to you, but trust me, it's insulting to them. If you buy a bike on the Internet, try to keep it to yourself and not annoy the local bike shop. You might need them some day. Tell them you bought the bike from your brother-in-law's cousin who fell on hard times. At least be kind enough to lie. And don't show them the big brown box it came in.

Another bit of truth, while I'm at it: your local bike shop does not really care to work on department store bikes either. They really don't. I really don't. If I can show you a pair of pedals that cost more than your whole department store bike (and I can), how well made is that department store bike, really? Cheap bikes are made of cheap parts, and cheap parts have problems right from the start. The threads on all of the nuts and bolts are soft and poorly formed. The metals used are prone to rust and fatigue, and things are easily stripped and broken.

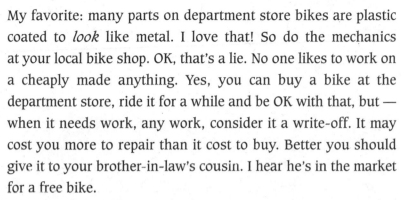

My favorite: many parts on department store bikes are plastic coated to *look* like metal. I love that! So do the mechanics at your local bike shop. OK, that's a lie. No one likes to work on a cheaply made anything. Yes, you can buy a bike at the department store, ride it for a while and be OK with that, but — when it needs work, any work, consider it a write-off. It may cost you more to repair than it cost to buy. Better you should give it to your brother-in-law's cousin. I hear he's in the market for a free bike.

Big News Flash Here: you don't have to buy new, you know. You could buy a used bike. Really? Yes, really. I have. So could you. Of course, you need to know that buying used adds a certain level of adventure to an otherwise straight-forward purchase. Now you have to wonder what happened to that bike before you came along. Is it OK? Was it abused? Where has it been? What has it seen? Will it respect me in the morning? Will it even want to ride with me next week?

Generally speaking, the big advantage of buying used is that you can get a better bike for your money than buying new. Yes, you're buying an older bike, but that's OK. Bikes don't age like cars. Or cheese, for that matter. Better bikes usually get better service, and the better parts last a good deal better. Feel better? Good. The first place you should look for a used bike is, big shock here, your local bike shop. You knew I was going to say that, didn't you? Most bike shops will take bikes they have sold new back in trade from customers who come in to upgrade to an even better bike later. This gives you the chance to buy a nice bike at a nice price *and* get the backing of a real bike shop for that bike. It's a win-win situation all around. I would say, call around first and see which shops do offer second-hand sales. They all *should*, but I'm not sure they all *do*. It pays to call ahead, and when you do, mention my name. That should be good for a giggle.

Needless to say, department stores do not handle used bikes. Not a problem. Prime sources for used bikes in my part of the world are pawn shops and thrift stores. Thrift stores sell all manner of used merchandise that people donate, and at least a part of the purchase price you pay is usually going to some good cause. The pawn shop, on the other hand, is in it to make money, so the prices there are somewhat higher. Still, I've bought several bikes at pawn shops over the years. The little English folding bike I ride to work almost every day came from a pawn shop, and I consider myself very lucky to have bought it, no matter what the price. (It wasn't that bad, price-wise.)

And about that price: when you are shopping for a used bike, you have to know what you're looking at and what it's worth. Not all pawn shops and thrift stores know what their merchandise is really worth, and that can cut both ways: you might get a real deal on an expensive bike for next to nothing — or you could easily pay far too much for a bike that simply is not worth the sack it was bagged in. Before you go shopping for used bikes, price new bikes. Learn what bicycles in your part of the world come from bicycle shops and what bicycles come from department stores. Make yourself a list, if you have to, to carry with you when you go used-bike shopping, show-ing what brands came from where. Try to not get all excited and buy the first cheap bike you see. There might be a good reason no one else has bought that bike. Remember what I said about getting department store bikes worked on. That holds true no matter where you bought it.

Of course, you don't have to buy your bicycle in a store. There are other options. On any warm, sunny weekend, it's easy to find people having yard sales, garage sales, or estate sales. They are all the same thing: someone decides they have too much stuff, and throws a few things outside with prices on them. You come along, look over their junk and decide if you want to add their junk to your junk — for a later yard sale over at your place. That's usually how it works. Needless to say, this takes "Buyer beware" to a whole new level. Now you're not even dealing with a store, but just some family down the street. You will not be given a receipt for your purchase. No 30-day guarantee. No refunds. All sales are final. Thank you and have a nice day. Risky, yes, but again, if you know what you're buying, there are deals to be had. I will say this about buying any second-hand bike, no matter where you find it: if you see one you like, *buy it now*. Do not hes-itate. Do not wait. Do not mull it over. Buy it. It will not be there when you come back. It may not be there if you blink. When you see the bike you want — and you will know it when you do — *buy it*. Period.

You can also buy used bikes from ads in the local newspaper or from well-meaning friends. From total strangers, even. All the same rules apply: know what you're buying, know what you're paying — and as always, buyer beware. (That would be you.) That real deal can look real bad when you get the bike home and find that it was not, in fact, the fine machine you were led to believe it was. Too late. It's yours now. All you can do now is make the best of it and ride the bike until it's time for your own yard sale. Just make sure you put an even lower price on it so it sells.

If you are looking for the best deal on a bicycle, how about *free*? Does *free* work for you? I thought it might. (Works for me, too.) At least two of the bikes I own have come off of neighborhood trash piles on trash pick-up day, and one bike — one of my all-time favorites — I literally found in a ditch. Now do keep in mind that these bikes all needed extensive work. Two out of these three needed total, and I mean *total* rebuilds — down to the bare metal and back again. But still, when they were done, they were great bikes, completely rideable and fine additions to the collection. (That third bike only needed new handlebars, tires and a better seat. Such a deal!) Free bikes are like free money: how can you pass them up?

So how do you score a free bike? Well, it helps to know when the trash gets picked up. After that, it's all about luck and being there. JoAnn and I usually go out walking in the evenings after dinner, and we do joke about Wednesdays being Trash Night, as it gets picked up in our neighborhood on Thursdays. By late Wednesday evening, there are piles of who knows what all out by the curbs up and down every street. You never know what you might find — sometimes, you find bikes. Woo-hoo!

Early one morning, on the way to work (on my bicycle, of course), I rolled passed a massive trash pile miles from home (and miles from work). Just barely sticking out of the pile was the end of a bicycle fender. I stopped. I looked. I was amazed. I dragged the bike out from under the pile, left it there and pedaled

(faster) to work. The first thing I did at work was call my lovely, understanding wife and plead for her to drive over and
throw that bike in the back of our truck. She did, and after a
total rebuild, I have a beautiful and uncommon bicycle that
amazes all who see it. Did I marry well or what?

The Bike in the Ditch is another great free bike success
story. *The* great free bike success story. I pedaled past this bike
for three days in a row on my way home from work. "Hey, look
— a bike in the ditch." The next day, it was still there. "Humph,
that bike's still there." By the third day, it was all I could take,
and I could take no more. "Alright, you're coming home with
me!" In truth, the steel rims were so rusted it wouldn't even
roll, and it was too heavy to carry that far. I actually drove back
with our truck that evening and brought it home like that. That
particular bike has undergone two complete, down to the bare
metal rebuilds over the years, sports the first pair of wheels I
ever built and is, by far and away, the most wonderfully addict-
ing bicycle I have ever owned. It is the bike I want to be seen
on. It is the bike I want to be known by. And it came out of a
ditch on the side of the road. For free. You just never know.

The trash pile bikes and the ditch bike were all abandoned,
and if you live in any sort of urban area, you'll see abandoned
bikes all over. Well, I do, anyway. I joke that I have "bikedar"
and can smell them from three blocks away. Yeah, a lot of these
abandoned bikes were probably stolen, ridden until they broke,
and thrown down from there. Most of them were cheap bikes to
begin with, and many aren't worth hauling home. Still, every
once in a while, you stumble across a real find. How do you
know that it's abandoned — and that it's OK to play salvage? I

employ "Uncle Chippie's 24-Hour Rule of Salvage". That is, if the bike is not locked up and left in a public place, it's probably abandoned. If it remains there, untouched, for over 24 hours, it's probably fair game to salvage. I generally only apply this rule to bikes that have been obviously abused, neglected, and pitched. If they appear to be parked in a thoughtful manner and are in good running order, I leave them be, even if they are unlocked. I seldom find any really good bikes like this, but the junk bikes I do find get fixed up and given away.

And yes, it does cost money to get them back on the road. Not only do you have to know what a bike is worth, you need to know what it will cost to fix. How much are tires and tubes? What's it going to cost to replace that rusty chain? (And let me tell you: chains rust if you breathe on them. Literally. So don't.) How bad is that seat? Seats are not cheap. Neither are chains. By the time you buy a pair of tires and tubes, throw on a new chain and a seat, you could go down to the local department store and buy a whole new bike. Cheap, but new. Is it worth it? Sometimes yes, sometimes no. You do not want to know what I've spent on the ditch bike over the years, but it was worth every coin and then some.

These days, people are always giving me bikes. They know that I will fix them up and give them away, always at my own expense. Now here's the bitter, harsh reality: not all bikes get fixed up. They do not all have a happy ending. Some bikes, if they are too far gone, get salvaged for parts. Yes, those parts get used to fix up *other* bikes, but not all bikes make it back out on the road. C'est la vie. If you want to go the free bike route, you need to know what you're getting into, and what it might cost. Sometimes I think that all bikes — even the free ones — all cost the exact same amount. It's just that you pay the price right up front with the new ones and on the back end with the "free" ones. Used bikes bought get you coming and going. It's like they say: "You can pay for it now or you can pay for it later." Even if you find it in a ditch.

Which Bike? No, Seriously: WHICH Bike??

All right, enough of this. Talk's cheap. You want to ride. You want to know what bike to buy. You want more information than just "Buy the bike you want" or "Use the force, Luke." Fine. Here's the deal: almost every new bike out there works. As a matter of fact, you'd be hard pressed to find a new bike on the market today that *didn't* work for at least a casual ride around the block. About the only thing I can — and will — rule out right from the start is a high-wheeler. Yes, you can still buy them new. Feel lucky, punk? (And did I mention my interesting collection of scars from said high-wheelers?) As wonderous and graceful as they are to watch in action, and as wicked as they are to ride, high-wheelers do not work well in today's high traffic environment. (Sometimes they don't work so well with no traffic around at all. Just ask me.) Yes, they excel on modern smooth pavement, but it's the stop-and-go thing that will do you in. Or the turns. So: no high-wheelers, please. Are we clear on that? Good. Off we go.

And let me just say right here that the traditional thing with men riding men's frame bikes and women riding women's frame bikes no longer holds strictly true, by the way. Welcome to a brave new world where women quite often ride men's frame bikes, and I see men on what we have always called women's frame bikes because they appreciate the low step-over in the middle part of the frame. (Who wouldn't?) Buy the frame that suits you and how you want to ride, and don't worry about whether it's a "men's" bike or a "women's" bike. It's not like we're planning to breed them.

What does that leave us? Keeping in mind that this can all change next week, let alone next year, here's a rough list of the general types of bikes you'll get to choose from when you go shopping for your own: road bikes that are mostly about racing; touring bikes that look like racing bikes but aren't; mountain bikes that look really heavy but aren't; hybrid bikes that aren't as light as they look; town bikes that are probably about perfect (especially in town) ; urban bikes that are like town bikes, but heavy on the caffeine (Woo-hoo!); comfort bikes that offer a laid-back approach to life (not that there's anything wrong with that); cruiser bikes that are even more laid back (maybe too laid back?); recumbent bikes that are positively laid back and crank-forward bikes that split the difference. There are also folding bikes, track bikes, tandem bikes and trikes. Whew. OK, that's the short list, but do keep in mind that the bicycle industry might be ready to unleash a whole new category of bikes on the world as I type this, and that there are certainly sub-species of every bike on the list and maybe one or two I've forgotten to mention. Let's just go with what we've got for now. Here they are, one at a time:

Road bikes are typically road racing bikes, and for many that means bikes that are lightweight and super responsive, but uncomfortable to ride and expensive to purchase. Sometimes *very* expensive. Not usually considered a good first bike, but still, at some point, you should at least ride one to get a feel for what cycling *can* be like when price is no object. You won't believe how fast you can go. These bikes are seriously fast.

Touring bikes look just like road racing bikes at a glance, but offer a more comfortable ride, a wider range of gears, and more robust equipment to handle the rigors of long-distance touring. Don't be fooled, though: a good touring bike can cost as much as a good road racing bike, and is worth every bit of the money spent. This is the bike you want when you run away from home for good.

Mountain bikes offer tremendous stability, an even wider gear range, and (mostly) bomb-proof equipment. No wonder people have flocked to them for years. Available as full suspension, front suspension (hard tails) and no suspension (rigid) bikes, mountain bikes offer their riders a solid ride and no surprises. They work as well in the urban jungle as they do in the mountains. Maybe better. Complex, but not a bad ride.

Hybrids are half mountain bike, half town bike. A little easier rolling, usually with a front suspension, hybrids are a good choice for an all-around bike when you're not sure where you might be riding. They work well in modest off-road conditions as well as on trails, both paved and unpaved, and around town for errands and exercise. A good first choice to find out what you might like about a bike — and what you don't.

Town bikes are just that: bikes designed with the town in mind. Often featuring internal hubs as opposed to external derailleurs, town bikes give their riders an easy (usually unsuspended) ride on pavement and a low maintenance platform to handle errands and casual riding. If you were to only buy one bike and keep it forever, this might be just the bike you'd want. Of course, who can buy just one bike?

Urban bikes come with tattoos. I'm kidding. Urban bikes are a little bit edgier than town bikes. Sometimes a lot edgier. Often built as single-speed or fixed-gear bikes, urban bikes are responsive, low maintenance machines that reward their riders with a fast transit in place of mass transit in the city, but I have to tell you: they work well in the suburbs, too. (And only look slightly out of place.) Urban bikes are simple, fast, and very cool indeed.

Comfort bikes are the bikes for the 'burbs. Easy-going and easy to ride, comfort bikes are relaxing, not all that fast (by design). You buy a comfort bike when you've given up wearing a watch. Or, at the very least, you don't wear one when you ride. Time matters not. It's all about the comfort, right? It is on this bike.

Cruiser bikes are for people who never owned a watch to begin with. Usually sporting big balloon tires and that classic cantilever frame designed by Frank W. Schwinn, cruisers are the bikes of the beach. This is the bike for the late-to-bed, late-to-rise crowd. And I say that with more than a little touch of envy. These are not the easiest bikes to pedal, but the ride is unmatched for smoothness.

Recumbents are the weird bikes from Mars you see out on the road, with the rider just inches off the ground, all laid out on their back and flying down the road. Recumbents are fast and comfortable, but their visibility in traffic leaves much to be desired. For that reason alone, I have to say that they do not make a good first bike. Or any bike you'd want to ride in town and traffic, for that matter. But that's just me. I know people who ride them and love them, but I prefer the more upright, visible riding position of a traditional safety bike. Just my opinion. (They are fast, though.)

Crank-forward bikes are a cross between recumbents and regular bikes, offering a slightly recumbent riding position that allows you to put both feet flat on the ground at stops, but still get your correct leg extension when you pedal. They seem nice enough to ride and give you a stable machine that's easy to pedal. Maybe not the quickest bunny in the hedge, but this isn't a race, is it? If you're considering a recumbent, try one of these first. You'll be more visible in traffic, and that has to count for something. Quite a bit, in my book. (And hey, this *is* my book!)

Folding bikes are (usually) small-wheeled bikes that (always) fold. Great for inner city riding where tight turns are the order of the day. Perfect for smaller people (like me) who don't need a huge tall machine. By the way, it's OK to buy a folding bike because you like the way it fits and rides — and never bother to fold it. I never fold mine. Folding bikes can be had as single-speeds or multi-speeds, and at prices from "Great deal!" to "Oh, my!" If you've never been mistaken for a giraffe when you went to the zoo, try a folding bike.

Track bikes? Yes, you really can ride a track bike on the road, but it's skitterish and nasty fast. Also, it might not have any brakes. You should probably check that out before you ride one in traffic. Those same brakes that are illegal on a track bike on the track itself are most welcome close friends once you get that bike out in heavy traffic. There's one aspect to the track bike that makes it so very desirable anywhere: that fixed-gear drive train. Trust me. I'll explain later.

Tandems are the mass transit buses of the bicycle world, and the perfect ride for a party of two. They come in all shapes and sizes — and all prices. If you are intrigued by tandems — and you should be — just promise me this: don't settle for a cheap one. This is the one time that money matters, and cheap tandems do not do the concept justice. Spend the money for a good one. A really good one. You'll be glad you did. And did I mention that tandems are fast? They are — but you do have to work at it and practice as a team. Doing so pays off in unmatched pace and grace on the road. Tandems are cool.

Trikes are a funny thing. Literally, you can't not laugh at them. Still, it's tough to find a more practical machine for in-town errands and slow traffic situations. They do take a whole different mindset to ride, though — a whole different approach to balance — but trikes are a blast and if you have the room to store them can be a great replacement for your car. (Of course, if you get rid of the car, you'll have plenty of room for the trike, won't you?)

And Bicycles Should Be Made Of …
Help Me Out Here

Once you get beyond all the different types of bikes and trikes out there, you have to look at what they're made of. By that, I mean the frame. You can change out every part on a bike, but when you change the frame, well then, it's a whole new bike, isn't it? Bicycle frames are most often made of one of four different materials: steel, aluminum, titanium and carbon fiber. Yes, there are bikes made of wood and plastic and fiberglass, but for the most part, for the purposes of this particular book, we really only need to concern ourselves with two materials: steel and aluminum.

"Steel is real," as they say, and, by and large, it is the stuff that bikes are made of. I have never owned a bike that wasn't, now that I think about it. Strong, responsive and forgiving, it is also surprisingly light when done right and lasts forever when treated well. It lasts a long time even if you treat it badly, but yes, it will eventually rust if you don't take care of it. Oh, and that exotic "chrome-moly" bike frame? Just a fancy name for steel. That's all. Don't worry about it. Nice stuff, though.

Aluminum is about the only other material you might consider for a first bike, or when you get back into cycling after you've been way for a while. The price has certainly come down over the years, and aluminum frames are showing up in more models at lower prices all the time. I've heard people say an aluminum frame lacks the springy "life" of a steel frame, but I'm not convinced that argument holds true for all aluminum frames. Don't not buy a bike because it has an aluminum frame, but there's no reason to demand one either. As for the line about how they don't rust, that is true. They don't. They corrode, and that's just as bad for an aluminum frame as rust is for a steel one.

If you are in a position to buy a bike with a frame made of titanium, carbon fiber, or any of the truly exotic things that people are doing these days, good for you. I'm impressed with that, and amazed that you are still reading this book. It is not possible to buy a bad high-end bike. You can buy the wrong one, but it won't be a bad bike. I'll stick with the good old-fashioned steel frames. They've worked well for me over the years. I like steel. It's real. I heard that somewhere.

Once you get past the frame, you're talking parts. More often than not, many of the same arguments apply to individual bicycle parts. Steel and aluminum are the two main metals of choice, with titanium and carbon fiber for the high-end machines. By and large, aluminum alloy parts are a very good thing on any bike. They weigh less and rust less and work well. I try to not get too crazy about weight, but there's no denying the joys of a light bike, and alloy parts really help make it so. Using aluminum alloy for rims does help immensely when it comes to rust, as those rims are going to roll through every puddle in town. They also help you stop quicker if you have hand brakes.

Rims, brakes, handlebars, seat posts, almost everything on a bike can be made from aluminum. Exceptions must be made for things like bearings and axles and chains, but if you want to go wild, those can be had in titanium. It is, for a price, possible to make a bicycle out of materials that do not rust. The thing is, that would be quite a price. Why don't you just bring your bike in out of the rain? Much cheaper.

Getting in Gear — or Gears, As the Case May Be

After you walk into a bike shop and get over the dizzying array of makes and models — and prices — the one thing you're bound to notice are the gears. So many gears! Why are there so many gears? I saw a recumbent a while back with 40 gears. Who needs 40 gears? Not me. And I'm guessing probably not you. With the advent of mountain bikes in the 1980s, suddenly every bicycle had to have at least two dozen gears. I don't ride on two dozen roads. Do I need a gear for every road? Can't I use some of them twice? Why do I need any gears at all?

Last question first: you need gears because the human engine (your legs) has a very narrow power band. You are not the big engine you think you are. We bipeds like to move our legs at a set pace and strength. Within that range, we can go all day, but get us out of our zone and we flounder badly. And quickly. To maximize our ability, bikes have gears that allow us to pedal at the same cadence and strength no matter where we are. Uphill or down, the idea is to keep the pace. The more gears you have (theoretically), the wider the range of terrain you can ride. Obviously, if you live in very flat land, you might need fewer gears. I say "might" because there's always the wind, and the wind can be much worse than a hill. You can always get to the top of a hill. The wind can go on for much longer. And then blow harder. What fun.

I'm going to break gearing down into three major food groups: one-speeds, internal hubs and external derailleurs. With the entirely too obvious exception of one-speeds, both internal hubs and external derailleurs offer a wide range of gears on a single bike. The only thing you have to watch is this: if an internally geared hub has seven speeds, then it really does have seven speeds. If an external derailleur system says it has 24 speeds, it doesn't really. Or shouldn't. There are, on derailleur-equipped bikes, gear combinations you should never use. Remember ten speeds? In truth, they really only had eight usable gears. We'll get back to that silliness later. Let's talk about one-speed bikes first.

Much like Neapolitan ice cream, one-speeds come in three flavors: fixed gear, free wheel and coaster brake. Each has its advantage and disadvantage. If you live in relatively flat terrain, one speed may be all you need (but remember the wind). Here's a good test of where you live: do you always set the parking brake when you park your car around town? If so, you might need more than one gear. If you set the parking brake on your car in your own garage, you definitely need more than one gear! If not, let's talk one-speeds.

One speed is all you need ... maybe

Fixed gears: OK, look, I'm going to try to remain calm here, and not get all worked up. Who am I kidding? Fixed gears are, if you're me, totally worth getting all worked up over. Fixed-gear bikes rock. When the safety bike first came out as a replacement for the high-wheeler in the 1880s, it was a fixed gear. "Fixed gear" means the rear cog is screwed directly to the rear hub. No coasting. None. Not ever. You pedal forward, the bike goes forward. You pedal backwards and yes, the bike goes backwards. If the rear wheel is moving, the pedals are moving.

Always. This is direct drive and bicycling in its purest form. A fixed-gear bike is quick, light and completely silent. It also offers fantastic control at low speeds and climbs hills surprisingly well. If you want to experience the essence of cycling, you want a fixed gear, but approach it with caution. The addiction is total. When I say, "Buy the bike you want," and I rattle on about passion and commitment and desire, this is exactly what I'm talking about. For me, it's the fixed-gear bike that brings all of that out. Consider yourself warned.

One step below the fixed gear is the single-speed free-wheel bike. Still a lightweight and simple machine, the single-speed is a great bike for the casual urban rider in a reasonably flat city. Single-speeds require both front and rear brakes (where the fixed gear needs only the front), but they are still lively bikes and a joy to ride — and you're always in the right gear. No doubt about it.

Before I mention coaster-brake bikes, you need to know that it is also possible to get bicycles with "flip-flop" hubs; that is, hubs that have a cog on either side, usually a fixed-gear cog on one side and a single-speed free-wheel cog on the other. Sometimes they have the same number of teeth on each cog — the same gear ratio — and sometimes the free-wheel side is a little bit larger, allowing for a more relaxed ride and easier pedaling. If you're looking for the best of both worlds when it comes to one-speed bikes, there it is: look for a flip-flop hub. Now what about coaster brakes?

For so many of us, the coaster-brake bike is the bike of our youth. It is the bike on which we learned to balance and ride and be truly free. It is the Every Bike, and yet has become increasingly uncommon in our overly complex modern world. For those who need a quick refresher, the coaster-brake bike goes forward when you pedal forward, and stops when you pedal backwards. The brake is built into the rear hub and actuated by the pedals. This allows you to pedal, coast and brake all with your feet. That would explain the name. Yes, you can still get coaster-brake bikes today, and for many people, they are the perfect bike. Easy to ride, virtually zero maintenance, and usually reasonably priced, coaster-brake bikes are a great way to get around when the getting is easy.

I will say this: I have seen coaster-brake hubs wear out. Mostly, yes, through abuse at the hands (or feet) of a large, heavy-footed person, but they do, if you're big and bold, wear out. For the average rider (like you and I), they will last forever, and all you need to do is slap a little grease on the bearings every decade or so.

Ah, the joys of internal hubs!

Once you get beyond the one-speed bike — if you do — the World of Gears reveals itself in all of its glory. Or it gets really confusing. It could go either way. Before we plunge headlong into the snake pit of derailleurs (Can you sense my bias here already?), let's linger a bit in the happy land of hub gears. They know me there. I think you'll like it there. It's a fun place.

Back around 1902, the English Sturmey-Archer company patented a three-speed bicycle hub. To say this was a good thing would be a great disservice to a wonderful invention. The angels sang. Or at least hummed along. So did cyclists. Internally geared hubs are a wonderful way to get more versatility out of your bicycle without losing the simplicity of a coaster-brake or a single-speed drive. (And you can get three-speed hubs with coaster brakes.) Now you have a variety of gears to choose from, but without the muss and fuss of exposed gears. About the only downside I can see to an internally geared hub is that it does take a little more fiddling and piddling to pull that rear wheel off if you have to fix a flat or change a tire. It's a small price to pay for a wonderful convenience, and well worth the trouble.

From Sturmey-Archer's original three-speed, manufacturers around the world eventually got busy, and a hundred years later you could get 4-, 7-, 8-, even 14-speed internally geared hubs. Pick a number, and you can probably get a hub with that many gears. But how many do you really need? OK, yes, you only need one hub. But which hub? And how many gears? I have to admit, even with all that's out there on the market today, I still like the standard, old-fashioned three-speed hub. It has a lot going for it: it's very easy to use, lightweight, and about as bomb-proof as they come. The three-speed hub on my little folding bike is at least 35 years old now, and it rolls along silently and works as well as the day it was new. I appreciate that.

A true confession: about a year ago, I totally rebuilt my little folding bike, and in doing so, I built a new rear wheel for it. (I wanted rust-proof alloy rims.) The new wheel uses a Japanese three-speed hub — not an English three-speed hub. Blasphemy! Yes, I'm sure it is, but let me tell you: that Oriental hub is smoother than warm butter. Wow. And the funny thing is, it's about the same age as the original English hub that came off the bike. (I kept that, too, for later use.) Life is good. Life with a three-speed is better.

Just for the record: I do plan to bore you to tears with gear ratios a bit later, but for right now, you need to know that a standard three-speed hub means direct drive in its middle (second) gear. First gear (low) is 25% lower than second, and third gear (high) is 33% higher than second. That will all mean more later. I hope.

Needless to say (but you know I'm going to say it anyway), the more gears in a hub, the bigger, heavier, and considerably more expensive that hub becomes. A 14-speed hub looks like a bowling ball with spokes. That might be a bit much. I would, if it came to it, limit myself to a seven-speed hub, adjust the overall gear range to match my riding style, and be happy with that — if I weren't already so happy with my little three-speed hub. I do like the idea of an odd number of gears in an internally geared hub, as there is the assumption of direct drive in the middle gear, giving you as many low gears as you have high. A fair middle ground, it would seem. I try to arrange it so that I do most of my riding in that direct drive middle gear, as it would logically put less wear on the hub. Or so I keep telling myself. For me, so far (after all of these years), that still works.

Derailleurs and chain rings and cogs (Oh, my!)

So if internally geared hubs are all of that and more, why don't all bikes use them? Good question. There certainly was a time when more bikes did, and we may see that time come again, but for now, most bicycles on the market today come with derailleurs. "Derailleur" is a French word that means "to jerk the chain around with wild abandon and hope for the best." OK, not quite. But sort of.

Up until the 1930s, all bicycles seemed to get by with just one cog on the rear wheel. They might have had multiple gears within that hub, but just one cog drove the rear wheel. Then Tullio Campagnolo came along and figured out how to derail the chain as it flowed from the pedal-driven chain ring back to the rear wheel. The angels did not sing, but maybe they smiled a little, and certainly appreciated Tullio's craftsmanship. To this day, Campagnolo enjoys the reputation of producing the finest bicycle components on planet earth. Whether they actually do or not would be a rousing topic for a panel discussion, but for an old-school bike guy like me, Campy parts are the best.

So Campagnolo figured out how to derail the chain, and derailleurs were born. Initially built for racing bikes, and originally only for the rear wheel, the idea certainly caught on and now, if you walk into any bike shop in town, it seems as though 99.99% of the bikes on the sales floor are equipped with Tullio's little gem. Not his brand, mind you, but his idea. I suspect this has more to do with price than anything else. It must be cheaper to build a bike with derailleurs, cogs and chain rings than it is to add an internally geared hub. It also has to be something of an ego/advertising thing as well: I've got *ten speeds*! (As opposed to, say, just three.) Never mind that a ten-speed only works (or should only be ridden) in eight of those gear combinations at best — and let's not quibble about whether or not the rider knows *why* they have ten speeds, or when to use which one. Trivia. Mere trivia. (We'll talk about the why's and when's of all of those gears in a minute.) With today's triple chain rings and nine-speed rear cog clusters, 27-speeds are now all the rage, and 30 is entirely possible. Like I said, I saw a 40-speed recumbent a while back, and it would be, I suppose, theoretically possible to mate that 40-speed drive system to a 14-speed internally geared hub for, let's see, carry the two … 560 gears. Oh Daddy, buy me that one! Or maybe not. Maybe it's not the total number of gears you have that's important, but having the right gears for where you're riding. Could it be that simple? Yes of course it could. And it is.

For me, the biggest drawback to derailleur-equipped bikes, aside from being so maddeningly difficult to spell, is the idea that all of those gears and changers are right out there in the weather, exposed to the elements as well as any road hazard that might choose to reach up and hit them. Just keeping the chain rust-free is tough enough, but now you have all of those rear cogs out there, and the exposed mechanisms of at least one, and more often two, derailleurs. In spite of my aversion to them, I do own several derailleur-equipped bikes, including at least one with some of Tullio's finest work. He did a very good job, and all of my derailleur-equipped bikes shift well enough and are a joy to ride. They just get a little grungy, that's all.

Let's talk math — let's talk gears!

In this book, I'm trying really hard to use an easy-to-understand low-tech approach to bicycling, and so far, that's worked out. (At least, I *think* it has.) (Has it?) There are, however, a few technical things I'm going to have to say, so bear with me.

I'll try to make this as painless as possible, but it has to be said. Here goes:

When it comes to how a bicycle is geared, you need to know that lower is, quite often, better. Of course, to know that, you need to know "What is low?" You will also need to know how bicycle gearing is figured — and how you can figure (and change) the gearing on your own bike to make it more comfortable to pedal. And that, as you might imagine, means going to lower gears.

Just as cars are so often equipped with wildly optimistic speedometers showing velocities the car could never reach (even if you drove it off a cliff), so too are bicycles equipped with high gears you might never use — and will probably never need. Some bicycle manufacturers are finally getting away from that trend, but it's up to you and me to check our own gearing, and to adjust it accordingly.

The gear ratios on a bicycle in my part of the world are expressed in "gear inches". If you live in the metric part of the world, the conversion is easy enough. We'll make it work. The whole process goes back to when high-wheelers ruled the road: converting your new bike to old gear inches means showing what size high-wheeler it would be. It's archaic, but it works.

And it works like this: you divide the number of teeth on the cog on the rear wheel into the number of teeth on the front chain ring up by the pedals, and multiply the resulting number by your wheel size in inches. Fairly simple. Let's give it a try: if you have a rear cog of 20 teeth and a chain ring of 40 teeth and Johnny has six apples ... no, wait. Twenty into 40 gives you "two", so you multiply your wheel size by two to get the gear inches for that combination. If you have 26" wheels on your bicycle, you have a gearing of 52, and that's not so bad. For most average around-town bikes, especially one-speed bikes, 50 is a good gear to aim for. If you have metric 700 wheels (which are very close to 27" wheels), you can multiply by 27 to get your gear inches.

There are, of course, exceptions. (There are *always* exceptions.) Bicycles with smaller wheels, like my little folding bike with 20" wheels, do better with proportionally smaller gear ratios. Conversely, larger wheels, especially with narrower, higher-pressure tires, can still feel good with higher gear ratios. In real world terms, that means the 44" gear on my folding bike with 20" wheels feels about the same as the 66" gear on my fixed-gear bike with 27" wheels, and the 52" gear on the 26" bike is not all that bad. Whew. And yes, it is all subjective. Thank you so much for asking.

For so very long, it seems, one-speed bikes all came with huge 85" gears. (Remember: fifty feels about right for most riders.) That was it. Take it or leave it. Most folks took it and put up with it, but you don't have to. It's very easy for a bike shop (or you) to swap out the small rear cog on the rear wheel for a larger cog, and in doing so, lower the overall gear ratio of the bike — making it much easier to pedal. This is what we call "a good idea." But why? It all has to do with the human engine.

So what's with all the gears here?

We humans are marvelously adaptable, but honestly, we're not all that powerful. We can walk all day, but maybe not run all day. We can offer a modest power output for a long period of time, or really push it for a little bit. Your choice there. In cycling, it is better to spin a smaller gear and go further, longer and with less effort. Go fast (in a larger gear) and you soon run out of breath — and energy. To get more out of the human engine, many bicycles are equipped with multiple gears, allowing that human engine to work at a comfortable constant pace, or leg cadence. It's all about the spin, and spin is good. You want to spin. Especially your legs.

The whole idea is for you to be able to spin your legs at 90 rpm all day long, uphill or down, no matter what — into the wind or away from the dog. Ninety revolutions per minute, constantly. Yes, you could do more. (I'm comfortable at about a hundred, but that's just me.) You can also do a lot less, but anything under about 60 rpm is lugging and can be a real pain in the knees, especially uphill. The goal is to keep your legs moving at 90 rpm, which translates to one and a half revolutions per leg per second. You can count them as you ride to see how you're doing. (But remember to watch where you're going, too.)

It works kind of like this: you start out on level ground in, let's say, a 50" gear, spinning your legs merrily along at 90 rpm. On level ground, that works out well. Fifty gear inches feels about right. Then you come to a hill, and have to climb said hill, so you shift down to a lower gear ratio — maybe something about 40". Ah, much easier! Your legs are still spinning along at 90 rpm, but yes, your actual ground speed is somewhat diminished. You're going slower, but it's just as easy as pedaling on level ground. That's the whole point of having gears. If the hill gets steeper still, you might want to downshift again (unless you have a three-speed, in which case you're done for) to something like a 25" gear — a really low gear. Your legs are still doing that magical 90 rpm, but now you're moving along at barely above a walking pace. But that's OK, you're still pedaling! You're not walking! Well, not yet, anyway. I've got a 19" low gear on my touring bike, and I *have* met hills so steep that gear was too high. I have walked. May you only meet that hill going the other way.

Meanwhile, we just got to the top of the hill. Now it's time to work your way back up through all of those gears as your bike picks up speed going down the other side — but your legs are still spinning at that constant 90 rpm. Are you beginning to see why you have all of those gears? It's all about a constant cadence, uphill or down. Going downhill, you shift into your top cog — your highest gear — if the hill is steep enough. That could mean something over 100 gear inches — a *huge* gear. Spin that at 90 rpm, and you are *flying*. I have a basic rule: anything above, say, 60 miles an hour (100 km/h) and I stop with the crazy pedaling thing and just enjoy the view. Or try to hang on.

Now you know *why* you shift, but *how* do you shift, exactly? More often than not, shifters these days are either "thumb shifters" that you — get ready here — shift with your thumb, or a twist grip arrangement built right into the handgrip. Either way, yes, it does take some getting used to, and we all have to use any system for a while before we get comfortable with it and remember which way does what. It does take time to figure out what to do to upshift to a higher gear or downshift to a lower gear — and longer still to figure out what gear you're in, no matter what gear you're in. The one small advantage of derailleur-equipped bikes is that you can simply look down (and back) and see what gear you're in. That does help, assuming you don't run off the road doing so. *That* doesn't help at all. Most thumb shifters — especially for internal hubs — have markings on them to tell you what gear you're in; that helps, too. I still find myself, no matter what bike I'm on, trying to figure out what gear I'm in — and trying to downshift one more gear when I'm already in low gear. It happens to all of us. It will happen to you. It's OK. Shift happens. (Sorry. Couldn't resist.)

By the way: what do you do if you find a bike you really like, but the gears are all wrong? You change them! As I mentioned earlier, too many new bikes come with too many high gears, and never enough low ones. It's easy enough to change out the gears, but more often than not, when you do that, you have to alter the chain length as well. This is something I do all the time, it's not that difficult, but it can be messy.

If you have a one-speed or internally geared rear hub, it's easy enough to pop that single rear cog off the rear hub and add a larger one to give you all new lower gears. I went from the original 15-tooth rear cog on my three-speed folding bike to a 20-tooth rear cog, and every gear just got 33% lower. Ah, paradise!

For a fixed-gear bike or single-speed free-wheel bike, it's even easier. On a fixed-gear bike, unscrew the cog (don't forget to unscrew the reverse-threaded lock ring on the fixed-gear hub), and spin on the new larger cog. Single speed freewheel bikes take a special tool to remove the cog, but coaster-brake and three-speed cogs are often held on with a simple "C" clip. For all single cog bikes, you might have to add a link in the chain. Maybe two. This requires a special chain tool, so this might best be done by a bike shop. Beating the chain with a hammer does not usually produce quality results.

Changing the gearing on derailleur-equipped bikes also takes special tools. The rear cog clusters on these bikes are either the old-fashioned free-wheel style or the new-fashioned cassette style. Either one takes a special tool to get those cogs off the rear hub, but here's the good news: you shouldn't have to mess with the chain length at all. Still, unless you like buying weird tools, this could be a bike shop thing.

You can also change a bike's overall gearing by changing out the big chain ring on the front crank set where the pedals are. Now, this time, we're going for a smaller chain ring to give you smaller overall gears. In the back, on the rear hub, larger cogs give you smaller gears. (Confused yet? Don't be. It's OK.) Changing out the front chain ring is sometimes a more involved process, and unless you really like tinkering, it might be a bike shop thing. Depending on the parts used on your bike, it may definitely be a bike shop thing, as special tools are sometimes required to remove some of the more complex crank sets.

You may never need to change the gears on your bike. The whole point of the gearing is to make sure you can pedal easily where you are — or wherever you end up. Always remember that 90 rpm thing, and try to keep an eye on that. Are you spinning

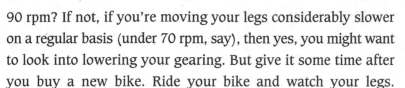

90 rpm? If not, if you're moving your legs considerably slower on a regular basis (under 70 rpm, say), then yes, you might want to look into lowering your gearing. But give it some time after you buy a new bike. Ride your bike and watch your legs. Ninety rpm. You can do it! Spin! Spin! Spin!

How Do I Stop This Thing?

Once you get going, you're going to have to stop. The faster you get going, the more likely you are to have to stop. That's life. To stop a bike, you're going to need brakes. No brakes, no stop — unless you hit something. So make sure you have brakes. OK, yes, way back when, bikes did not have brakes. They also didn't go that fast because the roads were awful and people were making the bike go by pushing against the ground with their feet. Today you need brakes.

You have a big decision to make right from the start: foot brake or hand brakes? This can be a tremendous source of anguish for many new bike riders, but it shouldn't be. Here's the deal: coaster-brake bikes stop when you push the pedals backwards with your feet. Hand brakes stop the bike when you squeeze the brake levers on the bars with your hands. Each has its good points and, well, not so good points.

Many of us grew up on coaster-brake bikes. It was what we learned to ride first and what we were used to for so many years. The coaster brake is simple and dependable and needs no maintenance or adjustment. You pedal backwards and it stops. Lovely. What could be simpler? Well, nothing. But maybe hand brakes are *better*. Here's why: when you stop a bike with a coaster brake, you have to keep at least one foot on the pedal to put that backward pressure on the pedal to actuate the brake to stop the bike. And if you have to keep that foot on the pedal, you can't put it down when you stop. If you take your foot off the pedal — to put it on the ground to hold yourself up — then you've stopped applying the brakes, and the bike could keep rolling forward. And that's not good if you want to stop. Tough choice there. And it doesn't help that it's usually a little bit harder to balance a bike at low speeds than if you're really clipping along. Not to mention those low-speed fall-overs are really embarrassing. I know that for a fact.

Hand brakes, on the other, um, hand, are not that hard to learn to use. When you want to stop, you simply squeeze both brake levers on the handlebars and the bike stops. This leaves both feet free to do whatever they want. They can sit quietly on the pedals, they can drop like sturdy landing gear to hold you up or you can wave them wildly around and make a spectacle of yourself. I do that all the time.

I know that a lot of bike riders, both new and not so new to cycling, are always worried about squeezing the front brake lever too hard and toppling over the front of the bike. And yes, it can happen — but you really have to work at it. To save yourself from a stunning nose plant, the first thing you want to do is make sure you know which lever controls the front brake. Is it the left one or the right one? It doesn't really much matter, but I like the right lever to control the front brake, as it leaves my left hand free to signal in traffic. (We ride on the right here.) The front brake offers more stopping power than the rear brake (because your weight shifts forward when you brake, giving the front wheel more traction), so it really is your more powerful brake, even though both brakes are physically identical. All you have to do is know which lever works the front brake and, here's the tricky bit: don't squeeze that one quite so hard as the other.

OK, it's really not all that tricky. If you grab the front brake like it's a slippery eel stealing your gold, then yes, it might get very exciting quite suddenly as the earth switches places with the sky. We don't want that. We want a safe, smooth, controlled stop, but promptly. That means you're going to have to practice and get used to just how strongly and quickly you can squeeze those brakes without feeling the rear wheel lift. It really does take quite a bit of effort, but in a panic situation, you're going to want to know just exactly how much effort that is. Trial and hopefully no error. Practice some place soft.

If that turned you away from hand brakes, let me tell you why you might want them anyway. With a coaster-brake bike, it is not possible to spin the pedals backwards when you are at a stop to get them where you want them to start up again. Backwards is the brake, remember? If your bike has hand brakes, that usually means that the pedals can be spun backwards with crazy, wild abandon — right up to the point where they hit you in the shins. This is a great way to build your vocabulary, but a lousy way to spend time on a bicycle. Try to not hit your shins with the pedals. It can really hurt. Still, being able to kick the pedals back to where you like to have them when you start off again is a real plus, and one of the main reasons I like hand brakes on my bikes.

The other advantage to that "spin the pedals backwards" thing is that you can always keep your inside pedal high in a turn as you lean. This keeps you from dragging a pedal on the ground in a tight turn. You don't want to drag a pedal, no matter what the turn. It's good to have that option to spin the pedals backward to get the inside pedal up out of harm's way.

While it's true that some bikes come with both a pedal-actuated coaster brake and at least one hand brake (usually for the front wheel), most bikes offer just one or the other. Hand brakes come in a variety of designs. I'm talking about the brake itself here, not the levers on the handlebars. (Although they do vary as well.) You can get side pull brakes, center pull brakes, cantilever brakes, V brakes, drum brakes and disk brakes. You can also wire a big stick to the bike frame and drag that on the ground to stop. Let me know how that works out.

Side pull brakes have their cable come in off to one side, hence the name. They have an undeserved reputation of being fussy to adjust, but the finest brakes in the world are side pulls. But then, so are some of the cheapest. They work well, and the good ones are real beauties. Avoid the cheap steel side pulls if you can. I have alloy side pull brakes on my folding bike, and I like them very much.

Center pull brakes — can you guess? — have their cable come in right down the center, where it gets divided to the two sides. Didn't see that coming, did you? For some time, center pulls were supposed to be, oh, so much better than side pulls. Now these days, you don't see center pulls at all, except on older bikes. (Like a couple of mine.) These are good brakes,

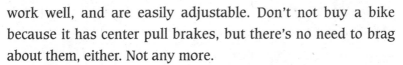

work well, and are easily adjustable. Don't not buy a bike because it has center pull brakes, but there's no need to brag about them, either. Not any more.

Cantilever brakes are the classic brakes for tandems and touring bikes where heavy loads need more stopping power. These brakes are built in two separate pieces, one mounted on either side of the bike frame, that together squeeze the wheel rim when you pull the brake lever. They work well, but if you aren't on a major tour, you might not need all of that mad stopping power. Still, these are good brakes. Great brakes, even.

V brakes are a variation on the cantilever theme, and feature long upright stalks that are pulled together over the top of the wheel to engage the brake. Much like the cantilever, these can be very powerful brakes, but they have also become very popular, which is a polite way of saying there are a lot of cheap V brakes out there. Personally, I find them annoying to work on and adjust, but that's just me. I'm a retro-grouch. I'm sure they're just fine. (We have them on our tandem.)

Drum brakes for bicycles have been around for a long time, and these days, you're likely to see a drum brake built into an internally geared multi-speed rear hub, actuated by a hand lever. You also see them in front hubs as well. (For years, drum brakes were the hot-ticket item for tandems because of their stopping power and the fact that they didn't overheat the rims as regular brakes do.) They work well, and seem to work forever. In theory, you'd think they would eventually wear out — like drum brakes on cars — but I've never heard of it. These brakes are about as weatherproof as you can get. If your bike has drum brakes, consider yourself lucky.

Disk brakes are the new kids on the block. They are the high-end hot brakes these days. I have seen them on expensive mountain bikes, but also on good tandems and some road bikes as well. They can be cable-actuated or hydraulic, just like the brakes in your car. They must work well, and should for the price, but in all honesty this is a whole lot more brake than I will ever need. If you like high-end gadgets, here you go: disk brakes.

Getting a bike to stop is probably more important than getting it to go. Brakes are that important. Maybe more so. No matter what type of brake you have on your bike, you want to be completely comfortable with it. You want to know just exactly how it will react every time you use it. I've seen too many people reluctant to ride a bicycle because the brakes scared them. They were afraid they would yank the bike to a stop and fall over. Don't be afraid. Brakes are seldom, if ever, that touchy. (People are seldom, if ever, that heavy-handed.) Get yourself on a first name basis with your brakes, and know what to expect from them every time you use them. Brakes are good. Knowing how to use them properly is even better.

Now Step on It! — All About Pedals

While it's possible to buy a hand-cranked bicycle with no pedals at all, they are rare. Made primarily for paraplegics, they work quite well and feature in-phase hand cranks, unlike the 180-degree out-of-phase foot cranks we see on almost every other bike. (OK, yes, you *can* put the cranks on a fixed-gear bike in phase and pedal it like that [if it has a cotterless crank], with both feet going around together like some sort of demented kangaroo. It's about the funniest thing I've ever done on a

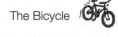

bicycle, but I'm not sure you'd want to leave it like that. [I didn't.] But I'm glad I did it just that once. What fun!)

For now, let's just talk about regular foot pedals. Most folks are happy as can be with the pedals that came on their bike, and very few run into problems with pedals that might require that they change them. The number one (almost only) problem? Sometimes your foot slips off. With the right — or wrong — combination of shoes and pedals, it is possible to lose your footing on the pedal. You can change your shoes, or you can (if you really like those shoes) change the pedals on your bike.

I'm going to divide bicycle pedals into three big groups: rubber block pedals, metal platform pedals, and clipless pedals. For the new or casual (practical!) cyclist, two out of three of these are going to work just fine, and the third will work if you really want it to.

Rubber block pedals are just that: pedals with big blocks of rubber for your feet. These are the pedals that came on every regular bike for decades. They are symmetrical, which means there's no "top" or "bottom" to the pedal. You put your foot on it, and you're good to go. For most people, this is all the pedal they will ever need. I had rubber block pedals on my little folding bike for years, and only recently changed them out. Good pedals.

These days, you are far more likely to find plastic block pedals on your bike, and these work well, too. They don't seem to last as long as the old rubber block pedals, but then what does any more? At least pedals are easy to change when they break or wear out.

Metal platform pedals come in a variety of shapes, styles and materials, from big BMX pedals to delicate-looking road pedals. (They aren't delicate.) They can be made of steel or aluminum, but trust me: you want the aluminum. Every time. Pedals tend to get splashed on a lot out in the real world, so the steel ones rust fast. Go for the aluminum.

Some years ago, "toe clips and straps" were all the rage on metal pedals. You don't see that much any more. Now, you either have a metal platform pedal or you have "clipless" pedals. Since I do almost all of my riding here in town, I don't need to use clips and straps or clipless pedals. I'm always having to stop and put a foot down. Yes, I know it's far more efficient to ride with your foot bound to the pedal, but I like my way better. I don't care to fall over any more than I absolutely have to. I'm funny that way. These days, I prefer aluminum platform pedals, and hold the clips and straps, please.

Clipless pedals are the latest thing in bicycle pedals. Essentially, they are miniature downhill ski boot bindings that clip the bottom of your shoe into the pedal itself, so you can pull the pedal up as well as push it down as you ride. This is very important if you're racing, but maybe not so important if you're off to the library. This system also requires that you wear only the shoes that have the little matching clip on the bottom for your pedals, and shoes so equipped may not be all that comfortable for regular walking. At least with the old clips and straps I could wear normal shoes.

These days, I wear any shoe I want, and often ride in sandals. The trick is to have good aluminum platform pedals that hold the bottom of your shoe or sandal securely in place

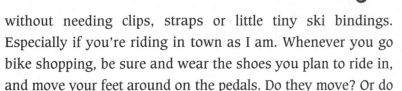

without needing clips, straps or little tiny ski bindings. Especially if you're riding in town as I am. Whenever you go bike shopping, be sure and wear the shoes you plan to ride in, and move your feet around on the pedals. Do they move? Or do they stay in place?

By the way, maybe I need to say something right here about the shoes I wear when I ride. I did mention that I ride in sandals sometimes, but, more often than not, I'm wearing shoes that do not use shoe laces. They use Velcro (hook and loop) straps to stay closed and tight on my foot. These are not high-end expensive shoes. They are cheap sneakers mostly, but for me they work, and they never come untied as I ride and get a shoelace snagged in the bicycle's gears and all. You might want to think about that.

For those who need to know, there are, generally speaking, three types of cranks on bicycles (four if you count a grouchy rider). The first type is the self-explanatory one-piece crank. It's just that: one big "Z"-shaped piece of steel with a pedal on each end. It's heavy, but it works well and lasts forever.

In many parts of the world, cottered cranks are common. These are three-piece affairs that use a nutted steel pin on either side to secure each pedal crank arm to the central spindle in the bottom bracket. Cottered cranks work well enough, but in the long run they are tough to work on, as you have to take the pins out to rebuild (grease) the crank, and sometimes that can be (warning: understatement ahead) a little bit difficult.

The solution to the cottered crank is the cotterless crank. (Seems obvious now, doesn't it?) This is also a three-piece set-up with a central spindle, but with this arrangement the crank arms are bolted to the spindle and easily removed, if you have the right tools. Thankfully, I do.

Odds are your bike will have either the bomb-proof one-piece steel crank or the more technical three-piece cotterless crank. Either works well, but I'll tell you the truth: I have examples of all three in my garage, and all three do well. You go with what you've got.

Does Size Matter?

And that's really the question, isn't it? Are large-diameter bicycle wheels really any better than small-diameter bicycle wheels? What? We're talking about bicycle wheels here. What did you think we were talking about? *Really?* Then this is all going to be very mundane for you, isn't it?

The arguments go like this: larger wheels roll over bumps better, but smaller wheels take less energy to spin. Narrow tires go faster, but wider tires are more comfortable. So if you had a bicycle with large-diameter wide tires, like the old balloon tire bikes of the 1950s, you could roll over about anything in comfort, but it would take more effort to do so. If you had a bike with small high-pressure tires, it would take next to no effort to move the bike down the road, but every little bump and hole would be a jarring experience. As is so often the case, it's probably best to settle for something between the extremes.

I have both. That is, I have the big balloon tire bike from the 50s and the sort of bike that uses very small-diameter high-pressure tires. If I were forced to choose just one, I would keep the balloon tire bike, even though, yes, it does take more effort to ride. There's just no denying that it is the more comfortable ride and feels far more stable on the road — or off the road, for that matter.

On the other hand, my little English folding bike has small-ish wheels, and it is a joy to ride. The other advantage of small wheels on bikes is that you can turn them very quickly. This is good if you ride in a crowded urban environment. Where I live, it is legal to ride a bicycle on the sidewalk, but you must yield to pedestrians. The folding bike is perfect for that and allows me the best of both bicycle worlds: both sidewalk and road.

I need to take a moment here and mention something: wheel size does not translate to how close you are to the ground when you ride a bicycle. I know, for many people, it is important that they be able to put a foot down quickly for stability when they stop. You would think that the bike with the smaller wheels would put you closer to the ground, but that is not always the case. The bike I own with the very smallest wheels is, in fact, the one that puts me the highest off the ground. Awkwardly so. My English folding bike, however, even though it looks almost identical to the just mentioned small-wheeled high bike is set up to place me several inches lower, making it much more comfortable to stop and put that needed foot to ground. About all you can do is measure the frame and compare the ground clearance. Or set the bike up correctly for you — the right seat height — and ride it. Does the ground seem far away? That could be a problem. Try another bike. There are many to choose from. Choose wisely.

Back to the wheels: whatever size wheels you end up with, they need to be something that is a common size for where you live. I'm not going to mention specific wheel sizes here, as what I see here as normal you may never have heard of where you live. Look around. Shop around. Make sure you know what size wheels are normal for your part of the world. That's the size you want to buy. That's the wheel you want to own. You want to be able to buy that much-needed tire or tube anywhere, no matter where you are.

Once you get around wheel size, you need to look at tires and their treads. Do you want smooth road tires or knobby off-road tires? If you do all of your riding on just one surface or the other, the answer is obvious. Smooth road tires don't work so well off road, and knobby tires are noisy and wobbly on the road (and are especially dangerous in the turns). Get the right tires for where you ride. It will make you happy and keep you safe.

The other consideration is tire pressure. Low-pressure tires ride smoother, but take more effort to pedal. High-pressure tires are tough to keep pumped, ride like rocks, but, oh, can you fly! As always, a comfortable mid-point might be the thing to look for. Harsh high-pressure tires can be annoying after a while if you're not in it purely for the speed. Very soft tires can, no pun intended, tire you out. (OK, so maybe I did intend that pun.) Look for tires between the extremes — they should serve you well. If not, you can always try something different the next time. Tires do wear out, you know.

A quick word or two about tire inflation: yes, you have to inflate them on a regular basis. I often end the stories I write about bicycling with the words "Keep your bike tires pumped" (those are, if you must know, the last five words in this book), and I mean what I write. Tires — all tires, good tires, new tires, any tires — leak air constantly. High-pressure tires leak air faster, but all tires leak. It's a fact of life. Tires go flat. There's nothing wrong with them, they just do. That means if you have high-pressure tires, you need to pump them back up once a week. With low-pressure tires, you can pump them up every two weeks, but don't wait three. Almost every tire I've ever seen has had its recommended air pressure printed on the side of it. Keep your tires, both front and back, at that pressure. No more, no less. Your tires will thank you, as do I.

One option you might consider is switching to "thorn-proof" tubes. These are much thicker and heavier than regular tubes, and might help prevent flats. I say "might", as no air-filled tube is truly flat-proof. These tubes are certainly more expensive to buy and harder to install, making them tougher to work on when you do get a flat — and you will. The additional weight is also noticeable when you pedal, as the wheel is now heavier, and revolving weight is more obvious in the wheels than the same amount of weight would be just on the frame. You have to make your own choice here. I choose to not run thorn-proof tubes, but I do carry a spare regular tube every time I go out and ride.

I've also experimented with the goo that goes in tubes to seal them, but found that when I did get a flat, it was almost impossible to patch the tube because of the goo. A lesson learned there. I'd say stick with regular tubes, hold the goo, and know how to fix a flat. (We'll talk about that later.) That's the approach that seems to work best for me.

By the way, those tubes for bicycle tires come in two valve designs: Presta and Schrader. Sounds like a comedy team, doesn't it? It's not. It's not even all that funny. Presta valves are the very narrow little valves that come on racing bikes, and Schrader valves come on everything else, including your car and wheelbarrow. Needless to say, you want the one that comes on everything. You want the one you can fill up anywhere without needing some special adapter every time you go to put air in your tires. (Which as we just found out, you have to do on a very regular basis.) So make sure you get Schrader valves. Don't listen to the argument about how Presta valves don't use a spring so you can fill them faster and easier. Not without the adapter you don't. Not even a little bit. Go Schrader. Trust your Uncle Chippie on this one.

Getting To The Bottom Of The Matter: The Bicycle Seat

Here is where we throw out all logic, a lot of common sense, and most hard facts. Bicycle seats are all about what feels good, and let me tell you: it's all between you and your bottom. While it would seem obvious that wider bicycle seats are more comfortable than narrow ones, that is not always the case. I have narrow seats that I can ride all day, and have tried wide seats that I could not stand for the first short block. It's not so much about comfort as it is about support.

The bicycle seat has to support much of your weight as you ride. You put a lot of your weight on the pedals, and some of the weight on your hands, but the vast bulk of … um, let me rephrase that. What very little is left is supported by the bicycle's seat. What this means is, the thickest, cushiest seat with mounds of soft padding may not be as comfortable as it looks. I know you want very much to think it will be, but it won't. You need a seat to hold you up and keep you positioned on the bike. And there's only one way to find out if it will: you have to ride it. More than just a little.

When you buy a bike at a bike shop, it pays to ask them about changing the seat out if you don't like it — *before* you buy the bike. Most shops are very good about that, but ask first. Ride the bike for a week before you decide. Just one ride is not enough to really tell if a seat is going to give you trouble. Sometimes seats can be devious little things that wait to turn on you when you least expect it. Ride the bike every day for a week, and if you're still happy with the seat, then you've got the right seat. If not, back it goes!

Just as you should never judge a book by its cover (except for this book, of course), neither should you judge a bicycle seat by looks alone. You just can't tell. Seats come narrow or wide, with short noses or long, and in any combination of both. The only thing I will caution you against are those odd "no nose" bike seats. Without at least a hint of a seat nose, it can be very difficult to control the bike as you ride, as we do use very subtle input with our legs to position the frame. So you might want to stick with the more traditional designs. Until someone comes up with something better.

And by the way, don't let yourself be talked into a narrow bicycle seat just because that's what comes on the bike or that's what "looks good" on the bike or that's what every one else rides or recommends. They aren't you. It's your bike. It's your bottom. So you put a wide seat on a narrow bike. No big deal. Are you riding that bike? Good for you! *That's* what matters.

Here's a trick question: do you know the difference between a bicycle seat and a bicycle saddle? There isn't one. I just like to call them seats (instead of saddles) because "seats" sounds so much more comfortable. There you go. It's all about comfort.

What else do you need to know about bicycle seats? Leather seats do take more care, but they can also, with good care, last a very long time. All seats wear out over time and have to be replaced. Sometimes this is obvious, but not always. If the seat starts to show a bit of sag, it's time to do some seat shopping. If it doesn't feel as good as it once did, here's why: it's time for a new one. Having a comfortable bicycle seat is a huge step toward having a bicycle that makes you want to ride. And if you have to throw a few more coins in the till to make that happen, those will be the best thrown coins you ever threw. If you ride your bike every day and never, ever, even so much as *think* about your bicycle's seat — then you have the right seat. Congratulations.

OPTIONAL EXTRAS ...
That Make It All Better

W E'VE TALKED ABOUT THE BASIC BIKE AND THE ESSENTIALS YOU need to go for a ride. Now it's time to have a little fun with that bike, and fix it up so it's just right for you. It's time to make your bike *your* bike. Let's check out the optional extras!

You know now that you can easily change out the seat for one that fits you better and pains you less. That should be done first. Get comfy on that bike, and you've got a good start. You can also change out the handgrips if they give you any trouble. Most grips are OK, but sometimes you run across a set that just doesn't feel right to you. Change them! Grips are cheap, and you can go a little upscale, get some nice grips — your hands will thank you.

The other thing you should consider is a pair of cycling gloves. These are usually fingerless gloves with extra padding in the palms. These are good things to wear when you ride. They save your hands from the constant beating on the handlebars and, should you ever meet the ground in a hurry, protect your palms from planet earth. These are all good reasons to wear cycling gloves.

Tingly fingers are a cyclist's recreational hazard. (Well, it's not really an *occupation*, now, is it?) You ride a bit and your fingers tingle or go numb. That happens when you put so much weight on your hands that you compress the ulnar nerve in your palms. This is very much *not* a good thing, and you need to make sure that it doesn't happen. You can do that by adjusting the relative position of your seat and handlebars. I'll bore you to tears about this in the next chapter, but for now, you should probably buy a pair of cycling gloves and wear them when you ride. I do. Every time.

Watch Your Head!

Let's talk about a touchy subject: bicycle helmets. I know, I know: you really don't like the way you look in a bicycle helmet. I don't like the way I look in a tutu, and it's kept me from a career in professional ballet. But this is different. You might actually *need* that helmet some day. (My tutu gathers dust.) There are at least two good reasons to wear a bicycle helmet, even if you never plan to fall off your bicycle.

First off, it gives you more visibility. That spot of bright color, up high on your head, is easily visible in traffic, telling drivers that there's a bicycle there. When you ride a bicycle, you cannot possibly have too much visibility. I try to wear bright colors whenever I ride, and topping my ensemble with a brightly colored or white helmet really finishes it all off. It pays to accessorize.

The second reason to wear a helmet is somewhat dependent on the first: the driver, seeing a cyclist in a helmet, now knows that you are out there on purpose. You *mean* to be there. It's not like you suddenly woke up and found yourself riding a bike — no idea how you got there. ("Hey, I'm on a bike! How did *that* happen?") You're doing this *on purpose* — and have the helmet to prove it.

In some parts of the world, you don't have a choice. You are required by law to wear a helmet when you ride a bicycle. Where I live, only children under the age of 16 are required to wear a helmet, but I've worn one for so long and so often that it feels odd not to. About the only time I don't wear one when I ride is when I'm on my trike. You might want to check your local laws on this one. It would be an embarrassing ticket.

I have four bicycle helmets. Don't ask. I just ended up with four helmets, OK? Three are solid white, and one is red, yellow and black. I wear one of them whenever I ride, except when I ride my trike. That just seems really odd, to wear a helmet on a trike. I may regret that decision some day, but it's mine to make. Maybe I need a special trike helmet, like an old-fashioned 19th-century British pith helmet. That would be cool. Say, I think I have one of those stashed away somewhere. Woo-hoo!

If you buy a helmet — and you should — please wear it when you ride. Every time! Here's why: if you buy a helmet and *don't* wear it, you're going to feel amazingly foolish if you fall over and you're *not* wearing your helmet. It will flash through your mind, as you watch yourself become one with Mother Earth:

"Say, you know, maybe I should have worn my helmet today."
Yeah, maybe so. Pick out a helmet you like and wear it. Please.

For me, having a good sun visor is as important as a good
helmet. Maybe more so. I know the sun will shine, but I don't
know if I'm going to fall over. The sun is a given, and a sun visor
is a must. Most bicycle helmets do not come with good sun
visors. It's just not part of the package. I've solved that problem
handily with Uncle Chippie's Plan B: I wear a cap with a good
visor under my helmet. It's just a lightweight cap in rip-stop nylon,
but it does a wonderful job of shielding my eyes from the sun and
cushioning my head from the helmet, making it all very comfy
indeed. Plus, when I get where I'm going, I can take my helmet
off and already have a cap to wear. It's a win-win situation all
around. So: good helmet, good cap, good ride. Good deal.

Fending Off The ... Whatever

Gloves and helmets go on the rider. Let's talk now about what
goes on the bike. Too many bikes these days are sold without
fenders, and for me, they are a must for the machines I ride
every day. Of course you want them if it rains, but they are
a good idea any day. Without them, it's all too easy to show up
at your destination all "skunk striped" by whatever you ran
through on the way there. And besides, you never know when
it might rain.

If you buy a bike with fenders, look for the full fenders that
really do cover both wheels. Short fenders may not do the job,
leaving you wet and icky when you'd rather be dry and not.
Obviously, you need them in the rain, but they also protect you
from any stray puddles, errant water sprinkler runoff, broken

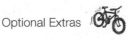

water mains, and my personal favorite: the predawn pile of puppy poo. Let me tell you: I was *very* glad to have fenders on the bike that morning! So look into a good set of fenders. They really help.

By the way, those fenders work even better if they have a good mud flap on the back side of the front fender. This is the extra-wide piece that will protect your feet — and shoes — when you run through a deeper puddle. If your fenders don't have a mud flap, I have made them from cut-up plastic milk jugs. They work great. (Mason St. Clair taught me that trick. Thank you, Mason!) Fenders are your friend, and mud flaps are their friend.

Be a Shining Beacon in the Dark — Seriously!

I have one basic philosophy when it comes to lights on bicycles: it is not possible to have too many. I subscribe to the Rolling Disco Inferno school of bicycle lighting. It is the law, where I live, that bicycles out at night must have at least a white light showing to the front and a red light showing to the rear. I have all that and more. We're also required to have a red reflector on the back, in addition to the light. (More on that later.) For now, we're talking lights on bikes.

Two reasons for lights on bikes: to see and to be seen. In an urban/suburban environment where you have street lamps lighting the way, being seen is far more important. The street lamps will show you what's there, but you have to show the drivers that *you* are there, too. I live just outside the city limits, where there are no street lamps, so I need a little of both.

Obviously, I use my lights at night. (Well, duh.) My simple rule is this: if I can't see the sun, I should probably be using my lights. That means on cloudy, rainy days I may add at least one blinky head light and a red blinking tail light, just to stand out in the grey. It's all about visibility — even more so on a grey day when everything blends.

In the beginning, when dinosaurs ruled the earth, I rode with a simple generator headlight and tail light, and they mostly worked great. Of course, they did stop working every time I stopped, and that was a bit of a problem. These days, you can get generator lights with battery backup. That's much better, but that generator is still a real drag. Literally. You do feel it when you ride at night.

A bit later in life (let's call it the Renaissance), I kept my generator lights, but replaced the generator itself with a big square 6 volt lantern battery that fit perfectly in a water bottle cage on the bike frame. It was huge. It was heavy. It worked like a charm. Let there be light! And there was, and it was good. Until the battery eventually died. Sure, I could have gone with a six volt rechargeable lead-acid motorcycle battery, but you have to draw the line somewhere. I eventually erased the line and started over with a whole new drawing.

Now, in these modern times, I ride with six lights. Yes, you read that right: six lights. Three headlights and three tail lights. All of them are LED (light emitting diode) type lights that work well, use little power, and can take the beating the bike (and I) dish out.

On the front, I use a constant-on six LED headlight that utilizes a quick-release mount on the right side of the handlebars to show me the way — and anything in it. On the left side of the handlebars, I strap a three LED strobe that really shows up and tells people there's a bicycle coming. I also wear a single bright LED headlamp that straps to my helmet. That one shows me anything I happen to look at as I ride — and I can look right at a driver and let him know: "I'm watching you, buddy." It works great. I've had people flag me down to ask me where I got it. I got it at a book sale (of all places), but you can buy them at any hardware or camping/outdoor store.

The same headband that holds that white LED on the front of my helmet also has a small three LED red blinking light on the back, for a high-mounted tail light that also shows up quite well. Again, this light moves around whenever I turn my head, and that's good — that makes it really stand out as I ride. I also run a five LED red blinking tail light that fastens to the back of the rear rack on my bike. Red blinky lights just say "BICYCLE HERE!" in a way that no other light can. You see them and you know you're looking at a bike in the dark.

My crowning glory, when it comes to bicycle lights, is the massive 18-LED red tail light I wear in the small of my back, held in place with a strap that ties around my waist. This thing began life as an electronic road flare, and was used as an in-store display in a bike shop to sell smaller LED lights. Forget the small stuff — I want *that* one! I have no idea where you might get one today. Try truck stops, I guess.

So that's how I go out at night and how I light my bike for my ride to work in the early mornings. The only sad confession I have to make is this: I know I really should be using rechargeable batteries, and I am not. Shame on me. Hopefully, by the time you read this, I will have grown up and seen the light. So to speak.

By the way, do you remember French arm band lights? They were all the rage in the big bicycle boom of the 1970s. I do miss them. Wish I still had mine. I wonder whatever happened to it? Ah, well. C'est la vie.

A Reflective Moment — About Reflectors

Just about any new bicycle you buy today comes covered in reflectors: a white reflector at the front, a red one on the back, reflectors in both wheels, and reflectors on the pedals. On some bikes I've also seen additional reflectors mounted on the bike frame itself. That is one shiny bike, and I don't have a problem with that, but reflectors are *not* lights. Never think for a minute that just because you've got a bike covered in reflectors that's all you'll need to ride at night. You need lights, and lots of them. Of course, all of those reflectors sure don't hurt. Keep them on the bike if you plan to ride at night. Maybe add some more, just for luck.

By law, around here, I am required to have a red reflector on the back of my bike at night in addition to the red light that's also required. (There's also a law that says my bike lights need to be visible for 600 feet, but just about any light is.) The thing is, that red rear reflector is a bare minimum for what you should have, if only to comply with local law. (And do check *your* local laws. They may differ.)

From what I've seen, both as I ride my bike at night and as I drive my truck at night and meet other cyclists, the reflectors that do the most good are the red rear reflectors, warning motorists that they are coming up on a cyclist, and those big reflectors that go in each bicycle wheel. The sight of those shiny revolving wheel reflectors can be a real life saver in traffic where cars are coming at you from either side. Drivers notice those two revolving reflectors, especially if they are out of synch, as they almost always are. Do, however, resist the urge to add more wheel reflectors. It's the odd loping pattern of the two reflectors bounding along out of synch that really gets the driver's attention. Add more wheel reflectors, and it's all a blur — and not nearly as noticeable.

Rear-facing pedal reflectors are also very good for getting a driver's attention, as they appear to move up and down as you ride along. That motion gets noticed, and getting noticed is good. Unfortunately, pedal reflectors lead a hard life, and are often too dirty, scratched or broken to do much good. Unless you keep an eye on them, they won't help a lot. So keep an eye on them!

All of those bicycle reflectors should be considered a good start, but not the end of all you can do with reflectors when you ride. I have reflective stripes on my bicycle helmet, I wear a very good reflective vest, and I also have pant cuff bands that are reflective. It's easy enough to buy jackets with reflective stripes built right into them, and you can buy additional self-adhesive reflective materials to add to your bike, backpack or clothing to make you more visible from all angles when you ride. I am not subtle about this. I look like a shimmering fool when I ride at night, and no one wants to bother the fool on the bike. I work that to my advantage. You should, too.

Of Sights And Sounds And Standing up (Wands, Bells And Kickstands)

There was a time, some years ago, when it was considered good form to have a tall fiberglass wand on your bike with a little orange flag at the top. There were also times when it was popular to wear polyester shirts and blow dry your hair until you looked like a Pomeranian dog in a stiff breeze. Thankfully, all of those times are long gone, and you don't see tall flag poles on bikes anymore. Fine by me. Those poles made it tough to get on and off the bike, you could feel them counter-sway as you rode, and I'm not sure they did all that much good.

Slightly better would be the short poles and flags we see in some locales that stick straight out the side of the bike into traffic, forcing drivers to make sure they leave you enough room as they pass. That, to me, is a much better idea. I'd be putting a sharp little metal spike on mine — but you didn't hear me say that.

The best idea by far has to be the classic bicycle bell. And no, I am not joking here. These things are great. I use mine all the time to give pedestrians a friendly warning that I'm about to run them down from behind like Genghis Khan in a foul mood. I'm kidding. If the Khan rode a bicycle, he'd be in a much better mood than that. It is common courtesy, and often the law, for a cyclist to give "audible warning" when overtaking and passing a pedestrian. For too many cyclists, that seems to mean screaming "ON YOUR LEFT!" as they go roaring by the poor pedestrian who had no warning whatsoever that they were about to be so adequately warned.

I take a different approach. I have a bicycle bell. I use it. I ring the bell, wish them a good morning (or whatever) and make sure I give them time to step right out in front of me, turn around, and offer me that amazed look of having no idea that they were, in fact, sharing the planet with other humans. Happens every time. Still, I ring my little bell, I say hello, and I hope for the best.

If you do get a bell for your bike — for the humor if nothing else — make sure you get a traditional-sounding one. You know, the old "B-B-B-B-ring, b-b-b-b-ring!" type. At least then they might have some vague inkling of what's about to run them down. Buy the bell. Ring the bell. But still pass with caution.

Just as so many "serious" cyclists wouldn't be caught dead with a bicycle bell on their handlebars, too many cyclists forego the traditional bicycle kickstand as well. Yes, it does add weight to your bike, and I will admit that I do not have a kickstand on every bike, but they sure do come in handy on the bikes that have them, and I think they are worth their weight for the convenience. If weight matters to you, get one of the light alloy kickstands. They don't weigh much at all and work great.

If you want to go a little crazy, get a two-footed kickstand. They are supremely stable, tuck nicely up out of the way, and hold the bike absolutely upright. That alone can make them worth the price when you go to load things on the rear rack. They are uncommon — you'll probably have to order it from your local bicycle shop — and they are not cheap, but they are worth it for the stability and coolness factor.

Most new bikes today come with decent kickstands, so you should be all set there. If not, a trip to the bike shop will fix you up in short order. Just remember, if you go to buy a kickstand for a bike you already have, take the bike with you. Kickstands have to be the correct leg length to work — and that length differs from bike to bike. Cut it too short just once, and you have to start over with a new kickstand. So take a stand — and buy a kickstand for your bike.

Making Your Bike Haul ... Stuff

The whole idea of being a *practical* cyclist is having the ability to do practical things with your bike. Usually, that means running short errands and carrying small things on your bike, rather than using your great big car to carry some small item. Especially if you're not going all that far. Being able to haul just a few small items on your bike will give you the chance to ride your bike that much more. And you do want to ride your bike more, don't you? I thought so.

I get by, day in and day out, with a medium-size yellow backpack. It comes with me every day on my ride to work. It's large enough to carry a small tool kit, rain poncho, my lunch, and the lights for the bike on the trip home. I like the idea of it being bright yellow, so people see me on the road. It's a visibility thing. In spite of that lengthy list of contents, it doesn't weigh all that much, and on my little folding bike I can strap the pack to the back of the bike and don't have to carry it at all. Even better.

If you're carrying less, a belt pack will usually do the trick. On my weekend rides, that's all I take to carry my tool kit.

Again, bright colors are the order of the day. Try to stay visible, no matter what.

Shoulder-slung messenger bags are very popular these days, and I have a couple, but I can't get used to them on the bike. They tend to shift and move as I ride, and usually end up sliding around towards the front to get in the way. Yes, they look very trendy and edgy, but that hardly matters when they slide around and stop you from pedaling. Unless you want to look good when you fall.

The key to success with any of these bags is to not carry too much in them. Travel light. Otherwise, they become an uncomfortable burden and bicycling is not the happy journey it was meant to be. If you need to carry more, there are other options.

Front baskets, both in wire and wicker, have been popular for decades, if not centuries. There's no denying the convenience, and the advantage of being able to keep an eye on whatever it is you're carrying. This would be the ideal way to haul a bag of eels, for instance. You sure don't want those getting away. (Or maybe you do. I would.) You do need to know that a front basket can be easily overloaded, and all of that weight right up front makes steering difficult, if not impossible. Again, traveling light is the word of the day. (Two words, actually.)

For heavier loads, a good rear rack is the way to go. These usually mount just under the seat and down by the rear axle and can be set up any number of ways. Most standard rear racks on the market today have a sort of spring-loaded trap to hold things in place. I hardly ever use it. I use stretch cords (bungee cords) and often a length of good old-fashioned nylon rope that I always carry with me. (Hey, you never know ...)

I once nearly ran over a sewing machine on my ride to work in the dark. I stopped, assessed the situation, then strapped the thing to my rear rack with that nylon rope. I think the sewing machine weighed more than the bike, but it was coming home with me! That bit of salvage was made possible by a six-foot (two meter) length of lightweight nylon rope that I carry for just such adventures. Go team.

It's also possible to fasten a front basket on top of your rear rack, and that works well, even if you can't keep an eye on those eels. Sometimes you have to trust them. On this side of the planet, we are knee-deep in big square plastic storage bins, and I have been known to fasten one of those to a rear rack as well. They work well, and can be had in bright colors to boot. Always go with the bright colors, even if they don't match your shoes. Be daring. Be visible. Always be visible.

It is still possible to buy the old-fashioned wire saddle baskets that were so popular back when your evening newspaper was delivered by a kid on a bike. Good luck finding an evening newspaper, but your local bike shop will have those wire saddle baskets just waiting for you — and they are a wonderful way to haul more stuff than you ever imagined, and more than you probably should. (It's very easy to end up hauling too much.) Travel light, yes, but when you can't, be ready to carry your burden in style.

You need to know this: sometimes I go a little nuts. ("*Sometimes*"?) ("*A little*"?) Hush. At one point, several years ago, I took one of my bikes and added wire saddle baskets — the largest I could find — to both the front and back of the bike. On top of both of those, I added huge wire front baskets that were fastened and hinged to the wire basket. You could pull the top baskets up out of the way, fill the saddle baskets, drop the top baskets back in place, and then fill those. It was massive. It was amazing. It was like a rolling shark cage. It was total overkill, and after a bit I regained what little sense I do have and took them off and built myself a trike instead. I still have all of those baskets safely tucked away in the garage, should the need arise. The trike, by the way, features cup holders in the cargo bed's tailgate. Still crazy after all these years.

By the way, "panniers" is just a fancy word for cloth saddlebags. You can get front panniers or rear panniers, but you've still just bought a pair of cloth saddlebags. They work great for long distance touring, but maybe not so great for everyday urban/suburban riding, where they're going to get scuffed and worn and damaged fairly quickly in the rough and ready world of practical cycling. I'd say stick with metal rear racks and wire baskets and you'll be fine. If you want, they do make folding wire saddle baskets that tuck in tight against the bike when not in use. Very clever, that.

Whatever your plan, it pays to have one. Even if you don't plan to ever haul anything anywhere, you just never know when you might ride over a sewing machine in the dark. And by the way, it worked just fine. Still does.

OK, Let's Get Serious — Seriously

It's a great big world out there, and not everyone in it is entirely honest. If that comes as a shock to you, you really do need to get out more. Or watch TV. If you own a bicycle, then you need to know that it is very easy to steal a bike. People do it all the time. Sometimes the same people, time and time again. It's that easy. If you want to keep your bike, you're going to have to get all proactive about it. You're going to have to lock it up when you go someplace with it. Every time. No matter what. Seriously.

Now, the thing is, you don't have to make your bike absolutely, totally, mind-numbingly theft-proof. No one can do that. It's not possible. It's like you and your friend being chased by a bear: you don't have to outrun the bear. You just have to outrun your friend. Similarly, you have to make your bike harder to steal than the one parked next to it. And you can do that. Just strap a bear to it. I'm kidding. (But that *would* work!)

Just as I always carry a length of nylon rope to drag sewing machines home in the dark, I also carry a small steel cable and a little brass combination lock. The cable rolls up tight, and the lock holds it that way until I need it. And most of the time, I can even remember the combination. (Beats searching for a key I would have lost ages ago.) Whenever I run an errand and have to park my bike outside, I lock it to the bike rack with this cable and lock, and that seems to have worked so far. Yes, a determined thief could probably chew through that thin cable in five minutes, but it would play havoc with his fillings. Serves him right. One of these days I'll get a longer, heavier cable and a bigger lock, but for now, and for years, this has worked well for me.

Part of the trick in keeping your bike your bike is not just that you do lock it up, but *where* and *how* you lock it up as well. If there's a bike rack near a high-traffic area — like near the store's front door — then that's what you want to use. If, for some wrong reason, the bike rack is around back in a dark alley, you do *not* want to use that rack. That usually means the store owner's brother is a bicycle thief, and you do not want to give them your business. Or your bicycle. Park right up front, where everyone can see your bike. Otherwise, it could be a long walk home.

When you lock your bike up, take the time to really lock *all* of it up. That means running a chain or cable through both wheels and the frame. I've seen some cyclists run a second, lighter cable through the bike's seat frame, to make sure they had a place to sit on the ride home. That's not a bad idea either. Crimes of convenience can be made even easier when the bicycle uses a quick release seat post clamp. Turn one little lever and you have a free bicycle seat! Woo-hoo! No, wait — that's bad.

You need to consider what you are about to lock your bike to. Never, ever, just wrap the cable or chain through the wheels and frame and leave it like that — locked to nothing else. That just means the thief will have to pick it up and carry it, and unless your bike weighs more than a small crowd of people, that won't be any problem at all. Be sure and kiss your bike goodbye if you lock it up like that. It won't be there when you get back.

Make sure, when you lock your bike, that you are locking it to a most sincerely immovable object. If it's in a bike rack, is the bike rack set in concrete? At least bolted to the ground? Chained to something else? If not, this is a risky lock up. If you lock your bike to any metal pole, is that pole truly fastened in place? There are such things as "sucker poles" that look like a good place to lock a bike, but are easily pulled out of the ground — for the express purpose of taking the bike that was locked to it. Don't be a sucker. Make sure you've locked your bike to a seriously stationary object.

If you have to lock your bike to a tree, make sure it's a big tree — one that would take considerable effort to saw down just to get your bike. Small landscape saplings don't count. Neither do bushes. Trust no one. Lock your bike to a fixed, heavy object. Let the bear eat someone else's bike.

Anything that you can't chain down, take with you. Just as that seat can be taken in a heartbeat if the post is held by a quick release clamp, lights, bags, water bottles and other accessories can all be lifted, filched, fingered and swiped so quickly no one would ever notice. Well, you will, when you get back. By then, it's too late. It's all long gone. Lock it up or bring it with you. Those are the only two choices that won't cost you money and grief.

By the way, do I need to tell you to *never* lock your bike to the bike rack sideways? Man, that's annoying! If you want to bother every other cyclist that comes along, go ahead and lock your bike sideways across the entire bike rack so no one else can use it. You'll make tons of great friends that way. Or at least learn some new and interesting words that you can use later if you ever take up golf.

OK, worse case scenario: make sure you have, safe at home, all of the records about your bike, should it ever get stolen. You want to be able to show sales receipts, serial numbers and all

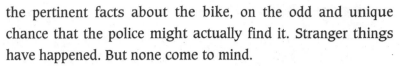

the pertinent facts about the bike, on the odd and unique chance that the police might actually find it. Stranger things have happened. But none come to mind.

Ride safe and lock safer. May you outrun the bear every time.

Tools Are Your Friend — But How Many Friends Do You Need?

This is not a bicycle repair manual. I told you that right at first, and I still mean it. There are, however, a few things you need to know about bike repair to keep your bike running well and to keep you riding. Little things. Easy things. You can do these things.

I mentioned bike tires, and how you should always keep yours pumped. That helps a lot. Keep up the good work. In all honesty, it's very uncommon for a bicycle part (any bicycle part) to suddenly break. It can happen, though, and you need to know what to do if it does — to get yourself home if nothing else. To do that, to ensure that you get home, you might want to consider carrying just a bare minimum of tools when you ride any further than you'd care to walk back. Bring your own safety net. You might need it some day.

When I go for a ride, I carry a small tool kit. I know, when I list this stuff for you, it's going to sound like a huge pile of tools, but it's not. It's all small stuff. All easy to carry. First off, I carry a spare tube, a small set of three plastic tire irons, and a little minipump. I make sure I'm always carrying the right size tube for the tires on the bike I'm riding that day. It would be embarrassing to end up on the side of the road with the wrong size tube. I haven't done it yet, but there's always a first time. If you only have one bike, you are quite lucky in this regard:

buy the right size spare tube, and you've no worries. Me, I have to check. Every time.

Tire irons are the smoothly rounded levers that are used to pry the tire off the wheel rim so you can get at the tube to either patch it or replace it. I usually just replace the damaged tube out on the road with a fresh, new tube. It's much easier and quicker that way. I can patch the bad tube when I get home. I have much larger steel tire irons at home that are easier to use, but they would be tough to carry every day on the bike. The little nesting plastic levers work just fine when they have to.

Of course, if you have no way of inflating that fresh tube, it doesn't much matter, does it? I carry an odd little no-name minipump in my tool kit that works great for inflating tires when I'm out back of beyond. I had tried some fancy (expensive) name brand pumps, but none have worked as well as this cheap little plastic pump I bought at a discount department store. I have no idea what brand it is (if any) or where it was made. I will say this though: try any pump you buy before you buy it, if you can. Absolutely try it at home before you need it on the road. Know how it works — and how well it works. If it doesn't work, get one that does. I went though a bunch before I found this one, now it travels with me everywhere.

By the way, I never did get all excited about those nifty little non-pumps that use CO_2 cartridges. I'm sure they work great, but I can't see carrying both the pump *and* the cartridges — and how many cartridges do you have to carry, anyway? And what if you need more? Too much to think about. I carry an old-fashioned manual minipump, and it works every time, no matter what.

Since the number one problem you will face on the road is a flat tire, you're going to need a way to get either wheel off of the bike so you can fix the tire. If your bike has quick release hubs, then all you do is turn a lever and the wheel comes right off — no tools required. If your wheels are held on with axle nuts, then you're going to need a wrench. I use a combination wrench that works on 14, 15 and 16mm nuts and was made to reach the tucked-in nuts used in the cotterless crank set, but will work on any axle nut. Any small adjustable wrench should do the job, as would any small locking pliers. I don't carry an adjustable wrench, but I do carry small locking pliers. They fit anything.

I also carry a bicycle multi-tool. There are literally dozens of different ones available on the market. Mine's just a medium-size one. It's got a limited set of metric Allen wrenches, some thin metric box-end wrenches, slotted and Phillips screwdrivers, and, of all things, a chain tool. The chain tool is a luxury. I can't imagine ever needing it on the road, except to win some bet as to whether or not I have one in my tool kit. The ends of the bicycle multi-tool also can be used as tire irons, but they are very wide and not very deep, so I've never tried to use them. No reason to. I carry a set of real ones. Real small, but real.

In addition to carrying the correct tube for the tires, I also carry a patch kit in a small tin. Yes, a real metal tin. Not plastic. It's large enough to hold a small piece of sandpaper to scuff the tube where the patch is going to go, some patches and a tube of glue. There are usually also a few coins in there, more for good luck than anything else. It's not like you can ever find a pay phone these days. That, in addition to the cable, lock and nylon rope, is what I carry in my tool kit. Enough to get me home every time. Well, so far.

I'll talk more about bike repair later on, but even then, the main thing you'll need to know is how to fix a flat so you can ride home. That's the biggie. If I'm just going around the block for a newspaper, no, I don't take my tool kit. And sometimes (Shock! Amazement!) I don't wear a helmet either. Shhhhh. Tell no one.

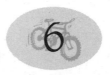

HOW TO RIDE A BIKE ...
And How Not To

ALL RIGHT, ENOUGH IS ENOUGH. ENOUGH WITH THE NUTS AND BOLTS, cables and locks, eels and bears and sewing machines. You can fuss with a bike until you are blue in the face, and all of that fussing will never be as much fun as the riding. Sure, I like to work on bikes — but they're a lot more fun to *ride*!

I am not a bicycle racer. Never really was. Oh, I time-trialed my tandem once. No idea what my time was. And I raced a high-wheeler once. Came in third — because the fourth guy crashed. That was all a long time ago, in what seems like another universe now.

I've done a bit of touring, but you'd never know it to look at me. These days, my idea of a long ride still gets me back home in time for dinner. Maybe even for lunch. And that's OK. I do put in my share of the miles just around town, going to work, running errands, and seeing the sights. I ride to work, ride to the store, and ride just for fun. Just for fun is the best, by far. You don't have to rack up huge numbers and ride for days on end. You don't have to go so fast that people hand you yellow shirts. You need but go, to your own places and at your own pace. As fast or as slow as you like, and only as far as you want. The bicycle can make a good trip better every time. It does for me. OK, it's time for less talk and more ride. Well, almost.

Get The Fit Before You Finish

You've got the bike and all the extras, now you are ready to ride — maybe. Before you go bolting out the door into the great paved beyond, we should probably make sure that your bike fits *you*. There are a few things you need to check to make sure you and the bike are the same size. This will help. Honestly.

The first test of any bike's fit is the stand-over. No need to over complicate this one: you stand over the bike and see if it fits. (To see if you fit over it.) What you want is at least a little bit of clearance between the horizontal top tube that runs from front to back between the seat and the handlebars and your private life right there above it. By the way, my wife assures me that this is not just a guy thing, but equally important for women. It has to fit all of us. No bike shop should ever sell you a bike so tall that you can't stand flat-footed over the bike and not feel that tube. If the tube intrudes into your personal space, as it were, the bike is too tall for you and that may cause problems in a fast dismount. You do not want that. Do not trust yourself to always wear thicker-soled shoes. That is not the answer. If you are buying a bike for a child, please do not buy

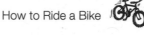

them a larger bike so they can "grow into it". They might not get the chance, if the bike is awkwardly large for them. Never buy a bike too big.

Now it's time for more of Uncle Chippie's wacky math. Lesson number two: how to get your bike seat the right height. I promise this won't be as involved as the gearing thing. This is one quick measurement, simple multiplication, and off you go.

Step one: measure your leg. Not just the inseam number on the back of your pants, but your *whole* leg, from the ground under the shoes you plan to ride in all the way up to your previously mentioned private life. The whole thing. Got it? Good.

Step two: now take that whole-leg measurement and multiply it by 104%. Or 1.04, your choice. The resulting number is the distance you want from the top of one of your pedals at the bottom of its stroke to the top center of the seat. That is your seat height.

Some things you need to know: this works no matter how you measured your leg; that is, it works with inches, centimeters, cubits or rods. You name it — any linear measurement system. The tricky bit is lining up the pedal. The pedal should not be straight down, but should have the crank arm — the thing it is bolted to — in line with the tube the seat is bolted to. For most bikes, this will form a nice straight line from just under the seat to the top of the pedal. It won't be straight down perpendicular to planet earth, but it will be a straight line, and the pedal will be its furthest distance from the seat at that point.

And that's what you're aiming for. If you have a bike that has the pedals set forward of the seat tube, you'll have to simply fiddle with it a bit to make sure you measure this distance when the pedal is furthest from the seat. Having a friend to hold things helps at this point, and your patience and persistence now will pay off with a very nice ride later. So will good math skills.

Now I have to tell you this: the first time you get on a bike set up like this, it might feel insanely clown-on-a-unicycle high. Not to worry. Make sure you keep that multiplied leg measurement handy, then lower the seat to what you feel is comfortable, but understand that you want to extend your legs almost totally as you pedal — and bend your knees the least amount possible. Your knees will thank you. You can always ride the bike for a week or so like this, then raise the seat slightly. Ride that for some time, then raise it again. Over time, that 104% measurement that felt so very high at first will feel just right. Trust your Uncle Chippie on this one.

The third thing we need to check is the distance between the seat and the handlebars. This is not such an exact science. There's no math involved. (You're welcome.) If the seat is too far from the handlebars, you're going to be putting too much weight on your hands. If the seat is too close to the handlebars, you're going to be putting too much weight on your bottom. It's all about achieving balance. It's as simple as this: put the point of your elbow against the nose of the seat and extend your forearm along (above) the bike's top frame tube that runs from

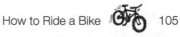

the seat to the handlebars. The tips of your fingers should just touch the back of the handlebars where they clamp into the stem that holds them to the bike. It's that simple. If your fingers don't touch the handlebars, you could be putting too much weight on your hands. If your hand slops right over the front of the handlebars, you might be putting too much weight on your bottom as you ride.

If you need to adjust that distance on your bike, start with the seat. By loosening the bolt that holds the seat to the seat post (the first bolt closest to the seat itself) you should be able to slide the seat forward and backward on its mounting rails in the seat clamp. That right there could be all you need to do to make this work. And if it is, boy, are you lucky! That was the cheap fix. Go team.

If that didn't do it, there is a Plan B: you need a different length handlebar stem. The handlebar stem, or gooseneck, is the part of the bike that holds the handlebars to the bike. It looks sort of like an upside down "L" or "J". See it? Yep, that's it right there. Now, the vertical part that goes into the bike is called the "quill," and the horizontal part that goes out to the handlebars is called the "throw." If the handlebars are too far away, you want a stem with a shorter throw. If they are too close, you want a longer throw. Fairly simple, no? Fairly simple, yes.

Now would also be a good time to look at the handlebars' relative height. Do they have you all hunched over? Do you like that? I don't particularly care for the hunched-over thing myself, but that's just me. Someone (probably older) wisely once said that you get to the point in life where you don't care to have your bottom higher than your brain. I'm so there. Been there for years. What about you? If the handlebars are too low, get a stem with a longer quill. If they feel too high (rare, but it happens), get a stem with a shorter quill. I like to have my handlebars about the same height as my seat, but what do I know? Sometimes it's all about taste and opinion. You ride what you like. Ride what doesn't hurt. And if it doesn't hurt, you'll ride more. Right?

One last little thing: it's nice to have your handlebars about the same width as your shoulders. Too narrow, and they constrict your breathing. Too wide, and you're back to holding yourself up with your arms. Handlebars that are too wide can be cut down, and handlebars that are too narrow can be replaced. I know this is starting to sound like an endless cash drain, but trust me: it's nowhere near as expensive as driving a car. Compare the changes you might make to get your bike to fit you perfectly to what you spend for a tank of gas (and how long that tank of gas might last). See? This isn't so bad, is it? There you go. *Let's ride.*

Get a Good Start — It's As Important As Getting a Good Stop

While it might seem odd for me to be telling you how to ride a bike, I've seen too many wobbly starts — my own and others' — to ignore the truth: not everyone knows how. Sure, most of us learned how to ride a bike when we were five or six years old, but that was then, this is now, and, well, maybe a few pointers are in order. Let's start at the beginning, or begin at the start. Either one. Your choice.

The safest, smoothest way to start off is to straddle the bike after mounting from the left. (Trust me on the left thing.)

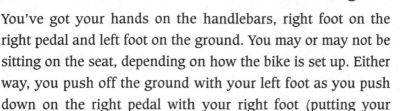

You've got your hands on the handlebars, right foot on the right pedal and left foot on the ground. You may or may not be sitting on the seat, depending on how the bike is set up. Either way, you push off the ground with your left foot as you push down on the right pedal with your right foot (putting your weight on your right foot), sitting down on the seat and hoping for the best. Do keep pedaling, by the way. That's important.

This is the wobbly part of cycling. Low speeds are the worst. Everyone has a speed at which they are comfortable and steady. Starting isn't that comfortable for anyone. Get yourself up to your stable speed before you stop pedaling. If you've started by going uphill, it may be a while before you can coast. If you pointed the bike downhill first, good for you — you'll be able to coast sooner. Either way, keep your bike above that wobbly stall speed. Your knees will thank you.

There is a wild alternative to the standing start: the Cowboy Giddiyup Start. This is where you stand on the left side of the bike (again the left side thing), both hands on the handlebars and your left foot on the left pedal. You push off with your right foot, then swing it up over the back of the bike as you sit on the seat and begin pedaling after the bike is rolling. I was never much for this kind of start. Too flashy. Even flashier: grab the handlebars, run down the street pushing the bike as fast as you can and leap on the thing as it's rolling right along. What's the one word I'm thinking of here? Ah, here it is: no.

Starting and stopping are the two times you're going too slow — the two times it's all wobbly and you have to be even more careful and watch your balance. Try to keep the risk to a minimum. Don't let gravity catch you off guard. Pedal!

Once you get rolling right along, you might notice that it's almost impossible to ride in an absolute straight line. You go a little left, you go a little right, and the bike sort of stays in a mostly straightish line. What you are really doing is steering into a continuous series of falls. The result is a gently arcing path, back and forth, as you ride. That's why you need a wider swath than the width of your handlebars to ride a bike. Three feet would have to be about a minimum width for you to ride in a "straight" line, allowing for the balancing arcs you (we all) have to make to stay upright. Don't worry about it. We all do it. We have to.

Let's talk about where to put your feet on the pedals. For the easiest pedaling, you want to keep the balls of your feet — the thick part of your feet right behind your toes — on the center of the pedal. Not the middle of your foot, and not your heel. With the balls of your feet on the pedal, you can flex your ankles as you pedal, and that will feel much better. There you go. You're welcome.

I wrote about leg cadence earlier in this book, but it bears mentioning again: faster is better. Not crazy fast, mind you, but a breezy 90 rpm is what you want to strive for. Why? Because it's much easier on your legs and knees and uses less energy as you pedal. That means you'll be able to ride longer and further with less strain and effort, and your legs will feel better when you're done.

If one of your goals is to lose weight, then you need to know that putting the bike in a very high gear and trying to push that monster cog is not going to help, just hurt. At best, all you will do, if you can do it at all, is bulk up your leg muscles and *gain* weight. You want to spin those pedals with the least amount of resistance to keep you and your legs thin. Spin, baby, spin!

It never fails: you get a good start, you're pedaling right along, and the next thing you know, you have to stop. I hate it when that happens — but it happens every time. (Unless you're on your stationary bike in front of the TV. Now there's a non-stop workout!) Stopping puts you right back in that wobbly zone where you can no longer balance the bike. The trick to doing this well — and looking like you know what you're doing — is to really stop when you stop. No hesitation. No second guesses. Brakes on, feet down, bike stopped. No bounce, no roll, just a steady, no-hesitation stop.

This is, I think, where hand brakes have the advantage. You can grab both the front and rear hand brake levers, stopping the bike quickly, and have both feet down for the landing. You've got it covered. With a coaster-brake bike, one foot has to stay on the pedal to keep the brake engaged. That's one less foot down for the landing. Yes, I do ride a coaster-brake bike from time to time, but I still like the hand brake idea. The landings are more secure.

Eventually, no matter what sort of brakes you have on your bike, you are going to skid as you stop. All it takes is a little sand or dirt, maybe even snow and ice. Tires can skid, and you need to know what to do if they do: let off the brakes! If you skid the rear wheel, the bike will tend to drift to one side or another. This is fairly easily controlled, and if you let off the rear brake, the bike will usually come back in line with no worries.

If you lock up the front brake, it can go badly. The bike will tend to flop right over, assuming you're not flying over the handlebars. If you're still seated comfortably and are still upright, it's time to ease off that front brake lever, and maybe apply a little more effort to the rear brake instead. A locked up front brake can cause problems fairly quickly, so you need to know to let go of that lever *fast*. At least ease off a little bit. The real goal here is to not get yourself in a situation where you have to panic stop the bike to begin with. That's the real goal.

It doesn't hurt to practice your stopping. You should be able to come to a fast halt and put a foot to the ground without that foot moving once it touches the ground. No slide, no drift, no rolling on and on — just stop, foot down and done. You can do it.

Turning Bikes And Missing Trees — All Good Ideas

The time will come when you will have to turn your bike, and probably much sooner than you think. Like before you hit something. Smooth, safe turning requires that you lean the bike into the turn. That means you lean left when you turn left and lean right when you turn right. How much you lean depends on both your speed and how tight you want to turn. Again, much like riding in a straight line, it's all about controlling a fall — and not hitting the ground. That would be the mark of a successful turn.

It's easy to think about this too much. Bicycles turn by "counter steering". That means that to turn one way, you steer the other way first, causing the bike to lean in the direction you want to turn. Then you turn the front wheel back towards the turn and balance your way through by controlling the lean. You quite literally fall around the turn. This can be very subtle, if the turn is gentle — or quite extreme if you have to dodge a tree that has suddenly jumped out in front of you without warning. I hate it when that happens. Trees have no sense whatsoever.

Much like learning to stop the bike quickly, getting the bike to turn is all about practice and getting comfortable with what both you and the bike are capable of. It's all about practice and knowledge. So practice. And know.

Remember our little talk about skidding? Well, bike tires can skid in a turn, no brakes required. All it takes is a little dirt or sand or snow or ice, and before you know it, you are one with the earth — and I don't mean that in a good way. The key to remaining upright, turn or no turn, is to be looking far enough ahead and understanding what you see, to avoid finding yourself in a panic turn on a slippery surface after some grove of trees has wandered out into your path. That means if you don't know what you're getting into, go slower. It's OK to go slow. This is not a race. It's all about having fun, and scars are not fun. Not much fun, anyway. Know what you're getting into, and turn carefully.

There's more to dodge out there than trees, of course. There are curbs and grates and railroad tracks. There are cows and snakes and possums. Animals first: be wary of farm animals — they're tough to predict. It doesn't hurt to get off the bike and walk past the herd (cattle, sheep, horses, whatever) if they are loose on the road. If you happen upon a reptile sunning itself on the warm pavement, do *not* run over its tail. It's not that funny to the reptile, and they can be surprisingly quick (not to mention venomous, so I won't). As for small animals like possums, if you slow down, they usually meander away no problem. And if you can't pedal faster than an attacking possum, you might want to consider bowling. Please *do* take the time to stop and move a turtle off the road and to safety. I would consider that a personal favor to me. Thank you.

I'm going to say more about sidewalk riding later, but for now, you need to know about curbs. If you ride on sidewalks, curbs can be a problem. Unless your city has gone out of its way to make each curb a smooth ramp for cyclists — not likely — you're faced with a vertical drop at the beginning and end of every block. It can be maddening. The only thing to do is to ride slow, watch carefully, and be ready to get off your bike at every curb. Sidewalk riding can be nerve-wracking. (But I didn't say I don't do it.)

City sidewalk curbs come in three basic varieties: vertical, smoothly ramped, and cupped. The verticals you have to walk over. Jumping them is hard on your bike and harder on you. (Not too bad if you have a full-suspension mountain bike, though. Do you?) The smoothly ramped curbs are a joy to ride, but tend to promote riding right out into traffic without looking. It's easy to meet a big car that way. Don't. Stop. Even for the smooth ramps. The new thing around here are "bump mats"; that is, mats that feature dozens of raised bumps at the ramp at every curb. These are supposed to help the visually impaired at intersections, but they make it a bit wobbly for everyone. Be extra careful on the bump mat. The cupped curbs are just annoying. They look smooth, but aren't. They can really throw you off as you ride over them and bounce you around without warning. Riding a bike with larger wheels helps, but not much.

One thing you can do to help get over cupped or steeply ramped curbs is to take them at an angle rather than head on. This works for going down as well as up. It requires a little finesse to do smoothly, and it does slow you down, but it makes the curb slightly less steep. It does help.

Far more dangerous are the storm water grates in the streets. These are usually big cast-iron grids set close to the curb — right where you and I would be riding. If the long slots in the grate are set in line with the flow of traffic, they can swallow your entire front wheel in an instant, leaving you face to pavement in the next. You have to watch every grate. Examine it. Know how it is made and installed. If you do find one that can eat your wheel, tell the city. Seriously. Make sure they are informed of the hazard. If it doesn't get changed, tell them again. And if it eats a wheel, threaten to sue them. Sometimes government only moves through litigation, or the threat thereof. Be very wary of street drain grates. They can surprise you.

We are, on the other hand, stuck with railroad tracks. They are not going to be moved, and even the very best of them can snag your wheel and play with it. Always cross railroad tracks at 90 degrees, even if that means slowing down or getting off the bike and walking it to get across safely. My brother once tried to ride his bicycle across a set of tracks that ran diagonally across the road. The gap at the edge of one rail caught his front wheel, threw the bike down, and left him stumbling along on foot — sans bike. He himself never fell down, but the bike was now behind him in the road. He was lucky.

Quite often, the pavement around the tracks is all broken up as well, leaving much larger gaps and holes than normal. Treat every set of railroad tracks as an adventure. They usually are. Oh, and watch out for the trains, too. They have worse brakes than we do. Better horns, though.

Bicycles And the Law — And Bicycle Laws

I've always said there are only three things you need to know to ride a bicycle safely: obey the law, obey the law, and obey the law. And mostly, that's true. Of course, before you can obey the laws, you need to know what they are. Find out. There are national laws, state or provincial laws, and local or municipal laws. Any or all of these may include bicycle laws. You really do need to know the law to ride safely. Ignorance of the law is no excuse. That's a law, I think.

In my part of the planet, we drive and ride on the right side of the road. If where you live did not get a visit from Napoleon on his last world tour, then give yourself a pat on the back and keep riding on the left. Either way, and this is *very* important: ride *with* the flow of traffic. It's quite probably the law where you are. Riding on the wrong side of the road, against the flow of traffic, is probably the second worst idea ever, topped only by trying to bring democracy to the Middle East. It's that bad. Ride *with* the flow of traffic. Every time. No exception. Please. I'm begging here.

The rules for a bicycle on the sidewalk are far more varied. Some places you can, some places you can't, and you need to know. Where I live, it's legal to ride on the sidewalk, but now the bicyclist is the same as a pedestrian. It's also far more dangerous for the cyclist to ride on the sidewalk as opposed to the street. Cars coming in and out of driveways don't see you, and you are traveling entirely too fast to be on that sidewalk anyway. Pedestrians will step right out in front of you, leaving you no place to go. At intersections, you are invisible. Sidewalk riding is mostly a bad idea, like just sending troops to the Middle East even without the democracy thing.

The worst way to ride on a sidewalk is to ride against the flow of the traffic next to it. Now you're just asking for it — and will probably get it in fairly short order. If you have to do this, be very careful, and know that no one is looking for you there. No one.

OK, yes, I do it. Even the ride-the-wrong-way-on-the-sidewalk thing. But I do it in places where there are very few — or no — cut-ins or driveways across the sidewalks and the alternative — the street — is narrow, busy and steep. Sometimes you have to choose between the lesser of two evils. It's still evil, though. Be careful on any sidewalk.

These days, I'm seeing more and more marked bike lanes on city streets. Mostly, these are good things. The only drawback I've found is, around here at least, that they tend to be on the busier roads I wouldn't take anyway and that the marked bike lanes don't get swept enough. They end up with a lot of trash and debris in them — and that means the cyclist has to go out around the debris field, that is right back out in the traffic lane.

There are also unmarked bike lanes — essentially just wide curb lanes — that get swept clean by the normal flow of traffic when there are no cyclists there. That works much better, but it's still usually a much busier road than I would normally ride. I tend to prefer the minor, quiet residential roads or bike trails.

Bike or recreational trails are the new big deal around here. Most of them are built along abandoned railroad beds and can go for great distances. Each trail has its own set of rules, and you need to know those rules if you ride that trail. Trails can be paved or unpaved, may be daytime use only, no pets, you name it. They can make up their own rules — it's not a real road. (Around here, bike trails are technically parks.) Find the rules, and try to stick to them. Some of these bike trails can get crowded, especially on weekends, and it pays to be courteous and obey the rules. That usually means going slower than you might normally, but that's OK. It's a social experience.

I treat bike trails as a sort of super highway system for pedal power. They get me close to where I want to go, then I branch off onto back roads and quiet city residential streets to get where I'm going. And it is comforting to not have to contend with all of the motor traffic for a change. Bike trails are nice. They get my vote.

Here's an important law you probably don't want to know about: no headphones. That's the law here, anyway: no headphones. Not even the little tiny ones. Even without this being a law, it's a very good idea. You really do want to hear all that's going on around you as you ride: the traffic, the warnings, the people overtaking you from behind, all of it. Sure, it's great to have tunes, but not if it's your last dance. Save the music for your rest stops. You'll be glad you did.

Do bicycles have to stop for red lights and stop signs? *YES.* Every time? *You bet.* Am I joking here? *Not in the least.* This is really important, and goes far beyond just obeying the law. This is about courtesy and respect. This is about life. This *is* life.

I have long joked that 95% of the bicycle riders out there ruin it for the rest of us. By going right through red lights and stop signs with no regard for the law or common courtesy, to say nothing of traffic, these cyclists give us the image of either ignorance or lawlessness, take your pick. Either way, we look bad. Don't do it. It's illegal, dangerous, and looks bad.

Know how to go through an intersection safely and legally. Usually, that means going through it just like any other (motor) vehicle. You wait for the light to turn green. You wait your turn at the stop sign. You ride your bike as if it were a legal vehicle on the road. Which, by the way, it is. Obey the law. Every time. We will *all* be glad you did.

OK, so it's the middle of the night, there's very little traffic, and you're coming up on a red light. Is that light going to change for you? *How* is that light going to change for you? Except for some new lights around here that use video cameras to change, most traffic signals use a double wire loop in the road to detect the metal presence of a vehicle. If you ride right over the middle loop, you might have enough steel in your bike frame to get the light to change. (Another reason to ride steel!) The loops appear as straight-line grooves cut in the roadway, right where a car would stop for the light. That's where you want to be — right on top of those grooves.

But it doesn't always work. The loop may not detect your bike. Jumping up and down won't help. All you can do is either treat the light as a four-way stop if there's no traffic coming at all in any direction, try pushing the pedestrian walk button over on the lamp post — if there is one — or, yes, run the light. Running the light is a total last resort, and not recommended at all. A better plan would be to avoid traffic light intersections late at night or early in the morning. That's what I try to do. Don't run the red light or stop sign in traffic. That's considered bad form anywhere, any time of day.

BEING A PRACTICAL CYCLIST — And That Would Be You

B EING THE PRACTICAL CYCLIST IS ALL ABOUT USING YOUR BICYCLE FOR more than just fun and exercise. It's about short trips to the local store, to the library, maybe even to work, if you live close enough. It's about getting out in the fresh air and under the full moon, rather than shipping yourself around town in a four-wheeled container. It's about enjoying the journey for a change.

So how tough is it to go ride a bike? For me, it's easier than walking. (You can't coast when you walk. You just stop.) I ride my bike to work, I ride my bike on short errands, and I ride my bike just for fun. And I don't have to ride that far to have fun. Quick, easy little rides are a joy, and any time I can ride my bicycle instead of drive my truck, that makes me happy. (A good day for me is any day I don't drive my truck at all, but that's just me. I'm still glad I have the truck when I need it.)

I will warn you that with the bicycle comes a sort of "cycle-think" — the bicyclist's attitude. As a practical cyclist, you will be more aware of the weather. You will not, as Dylan rightfully pointed out, need a weatherman to tell which way the wind blows. You will *know*, by personal experience. You will know every hill anywhere near you, both uphill and down, no matter how slight. You will know which roads have loose dogs, and which dogs are fun. You will meet people miles from your home, and they will be your friends. You will find small stores and cafés and places that you never knew existed when you drove by in your car. On the bike, they invite. And you will bore your friends to tears with all of this, but that's OK. You're a cyclist now. Welcome to my (very detailed little) world.

Fashionable Or Comfy — Pick One

Now I know what you're thinking when it comes to being the practical cyclist: you are, right now, seriously asking yourself, "Do I have to wear those slinky black stretch shorts I see all the other way too skinny people wearing when they ride their fancy-schmancy bikes?" The happy answer here is: no, you do not. I never do. Why should you? About the best thing I can say about those skin-tight black shorts is that they hide the grease stains when you wipe your hands on them after an on-road bike repair. Other than that, who needs them?

So what do you wear? Wear what you like. Wear what's comfortable. I go for loose-fitting cotton, but only because I get all itchy wearing wool. I prefer cycling in clothes that give me good freedom of movement, but without the stuff billowing out behind me like a parachute and maybe getting caught in the spokes. (So keep the Superman cape short.) I also like lots of deep pockets, so stuff doesn't fall out. Pockets with flaps that fasten are even better. Be comfortable. That's the most important thing. You can wear whatever you like. You don't have to wear the tight black cycling shorts. Unless you just want to show off.

Likewise with the brightly colored team cycling jerseys. Yes, it's good to dress in bright colors, but no need to go nuts about it and dress like a rolling advertisement for stuff you'd never buy. I do strongly recommend bright, solid colors, especially for shirts and jackets. Give the other people out there a big, bright patch of solid color to see — and maybe you'll be seen. It could happen. Shirts and jackets with any sort of patterns on them become so much urban camouflage, and that's the last thing you want. The whole point is to present other road users with an easily identifiable human form as you ride. ("Hey! It's me! I'm right here!") Keep with the big, bright solid colors to be seen on the road: red, orange, yellow, bright lime green, and even stark white are by far the best colors to wear. Pick *one*. And please, do avoid at all cost wearing any real hunter or military camouflage when you ride a bicycle. Too many people spent way too much time and money making those patterns invisible to the human eye. They were not ever meant to be worn in traffic. So don't.

Yes, I do often wear pants when I ride. (As opposed to shorts. Get your mind out of the gutter.) Most of the time, that means I have to wear cuff bands that cinch the pant cuffs tight against the bottom of my legs around the ankles to keep those cuffs away from the greasy chain and unforgiving chain ring up front while I'm pedaling. A small price to pay for personal transport — and wearing pants in public. Buy reflective cuff bands, and you've got that much more safety going for you, but wearing pants when you go cycling is OK.

Most of the time, because I do live where it's warmer, I wear shorts when I ride. I prefer the larger, looser fitting "cargo" shorts with lots of pockets, but any shorts will do, unless they are too, well, short. Short shorts are just a little too scandalous for me, but that's just me. No need for tight fitting special cycling shorts — I do a lot of my week-end riding in cut-off blue jeans. Just not cut too short. That's the long and short of it.

If I'm wearing shoes, I'm wearing socks. I never did get into that "sockless shoe" look. On the bike, and in shorts, I turn down the tops of the socks to keep my legs cool, but other than that, grey athletic socks are the order of the day. You sure don't require special cycling socks. Do they even make special cycling socks? Probably, but who needs them?

You have to appreciate any physical activity that doesn't require special shoes — and bicycling is all that — unless you have those high-tech clipless pedals; then you need the shoes to match so you can tap-dance your way through life off the bike. I don't have them, so I don't need them. I do my riding in cheap sneakers or sandals. I would say to avoid leather-soled shoes — too slippery. Any walking shoe or running shoe should do well, but heavily lugged-sole hiking boots might catch on

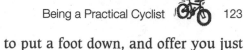

the pedal when you go to put a foot down, and offer you just that split-second of panic.

I do try to avoid shoes and sandals that use shoestrings. Shoestrings are too easily caught in the pedals and chain rings, and that can make for a surprising dismount. My shoes fasten with Velcro (hook and loop) straps and work quite well for both walking and cycling. If you do ride with shoes with laces, take special care to make sure the laces are tied tight and tucked securely out of harm's way. Maybe tuck them up into your down-turned sock? Just be sure and keep them out of your pedals and chain rings.

Mason St. Clair has long promoted wearing sandals when you ride your bike in the summer, and I have to say, as always, Mason is right. Riding in sandals is really quite nice in the heat of summer. They let your feet breathe. Now do keep in mind that we're talking sport sandals here that fasten securely to your feet — and not cheap flip-flop shower sandals. By the way, you know you're getting older when wearing socks with your sandals starts to look like a good idea. But you know, it is a very comfy combination. Uh-oh … does that mean I'm getting …? Nah, not a chance!

Wear what you want when you ride. You need not be a slave to cycling fashion. Be comfortable and be visible. Be happy.

The Physical Side Of Cycling

Almost anyone can ride a bicycle. You don't have to be in perfect physical shape. You don't need a body mass index of under 25. (Mine's sure not.) All you need is a decent sense of balance and a willingness to get out there in the real world and breathe fresh air for a change. You have to want to do it — and you can.

Will riding a bicycle get you in shape? Well, maybe. It depends on how much cycling you do. If you only ride a little and eat a lot, then no, bicycling will not let you shed the weight. If you watch your diet and ride some more, then yes, you might see the weight start to fall off. If you ride a bicycle all day, every day, then you can eat whatever you want and have seconds. Now bicycling is starting to sound like a good idea, isn't it?

The average cyclist, on an average ride, will burn about 400 calories an hour if they sort of work at it. Less if they don't, and more if they work harder. By watching your diet and cycling for a couple of hours a day, you should be able to slowly, carefully, lose weight — if that's your goal. For me, I've found that I have to exercise, walk, or ride a bike 10% of the day (about 2½ hours a day) just to keep the weight off. More if I want to lose weight. But that's just me. I don't ride to lose weight. I ride because it's more fun than almost anything else. It makes me happy.

Once you do start riding, two questions usually present themselves in fairly short order: why does my bottom hurt? And why are my hands numb? Let's start at the bottom, shall we?

Mostly, your bottom hurts because this is something new and you're not used to sitting like that or using your legs like that. By starting out with short rides, and not trying to do too much too soon, you can get used to the new bicycle seat and how you have to sit and pedal to ride a bike. Of course, it helps if the seat is the right height and is comfortable to begin with. I've explained how to get your bike seat the right height (104% of your leg length, remember?), but you also have to have the right bicycle seat to begin with, and that might take some trial and error. Every bicycle seat is different, just as everyone's bottom is different. (Not that I've checked out everyone's bottom, mind you.) I'm guessing here.

If after a week or so of riding, the bicycle's seat feels no better to you — or even worse — then it's time for a trip to the bike shop for a new — a better — seat. This is very much a learning experience for both you and your bottom. Once you get the right seat for you and your bike, you'll know it, and every ride will be a joy, if only you could feel your hands.

Numb hands are the second most common complaint for cyclists. The number one solution: wear cycling gloves. I can't stress that enough. I wear mine all the time. Well, whenever I'm on the bike. (I mean, I'm not a *complete* loon.) Cycling gloves save your hands when you're riding, protect your hands if you fall, and let you pick up turtles and get them out of the road without having to get your hands all icky with the slimy, wet shells. (Just make sure when you save the turtle that you hold it well out away from you. Sometimes I think they are nothing so much as one big hard-shelled bladder. I should have mentioned that earlier.)

If you wear cycling gloves and still have trouble with your hands, try checking the seat and handlebar position. Do the test with your elbow against the seat and see if your fingers can touch the handlebars. If they don't come close, the handlebars are too far away. Try moving the seat forward, and/or the handlebars back. This may mean that you have to buy a new, shorter handlebar stem, but it will be well worth it. After you get the seat sorted out and the feeling back in your hands, you'll be ready to *ride*!

Just don't go crazy. Start with reasonable short rides close to home. Around the block is a great start. Cruise around the neighborhood. Meet your neighbors. Stop to chat. Pet the dogs. Once you get used to pedaling where you live, you can branch out and stretch your legs a little. Ride to the closest store and bring back something you need. Ride to the nearest restaurant for lunch and back again. Start to look at maps and plot where you might be able to go safely. The key to success with this is to not try to do too much too soon, and to never do something that makes you nervous. Ride where you want to ride, at your own pace. Build up your experience slowly, carefully, and comfortably. Be the practical cyclist a little bit at a time, and before you know it, you'll be ready to go *anywhere*. Well, anywhere within reason.

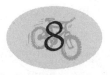

BUT WHERE DO I GO? ...
And How Do I Get There?

T HE NUMBER ONE WORST MISTAKE EVERY CYCLIST MAKES, WHETHER starting out on their first ride or being a seasoned road veteran rider (who should know better), is to plan their bike route as though they were driving a car and to take the same roads they would take if they drove to wherever they were going. Resist that temptation. It's easy to do. You've driven to that place a thousand times. You know the way. You know the roads. But you only know the car roads — you don't know the bike roads. While it's true that there are places only reached by one road, here in the city there are many roads that all, eventually, lead to the same place if you're willing to work at it. And when it comes to cycling, some roads are better than others. You want, poetically speaking, to take the road less traveled. It will make all the difference.

That means the first thing you want is a good local street map — one that shows all of the roads, however small. Many areas have local government agencies (like planning agencies) that offer these maps for free. Check with your local government first. Get a good map, pull up a chair and spread it out. Now, where do you want to go?

One of the first things you might notice, once you start to really study the map, is that too many of the small roads don't go anywhere. They don't connect to other small roads. In my part of the world, a man-made canal and a railroad line make a large "X" across the landscape, effectively dividing it all into irregular quarters — and stopping all small roads in the process. By the time you add a few major highways across all of that, my world is a series of stand-alone small road groupings, and getting from one grouping to the next takes skill, knowledge, and bravery. A little speed doesn't hurt, either.

Without having to use a busy highway to cross a canal, railroad tracks, or some other barrier, look at where you might want to go close to home. The library? The store? Can you get to work from home? How about a movie theater or restaurant? Look at the roads that branch out from where you live. Can small roads get you where you want to go? Is there anything in your way? There's a real sense of accomplishment when you plan a trip by bicycle, however long or short, and make it work for you. Most of the time, you *can* get there from here, assuming there isn't too far from here. Plan accordingly.

Of course, there's more to it than just connecting the roads and heading out on your bike. Are there any hills between here and there? What you need now is a topographic — or "topo" —

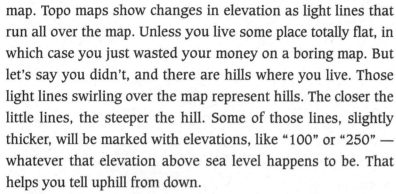

map. Topo maps show changes in elevation as light lines that run all over the map. Unless you live some place totally flat, in which case you just wasted your money on a boring map. But let's say you didn't, and there are hills where you live. Those light lines swirling over the map represent hills. The closer the little lines, the steeper the hill. Some of those lines, slightly thicker, will be marked with elevations, like "100" or "250" — whatever that elevation above sea level happens to be. That helps you tell uphill from down.

The goal, when you plan your route with a topo map, is to cross as few elevation lines as possible. Fewer lines equals fewer hills. Now, since you're going to start and finish the ride at home, they will, at least in theory, cancel each other out. In reality, you will always notice more up- than downhills. Life's funny that way. Just not the kind of funny you laugh at. Hills build character. Everyone says so. Just keep telling yourself that as you walk up the hills. That's what I do.

One way to reduce the elevation changes you have to nego-tiate — or at least to spread them out — is to follow a stream or river if there's a road next to it. Here, the slopes are usually more gentle. Yes, you are going either uphill or down as you follow the flowing water, but unless it's a white-water rapid, it's usually not too bad. Better still: go around the lake. Lakes are flat, so the road around them almost has to be, right? Well, mostly yes. It's a good start, anyway. Use the topo map to your advantage.

Once you get beyond which roads connect where and the hills between here and there, what else do you need to think about when you plan a bicycle route? Time of day can make the difference between a good ride and a not so great ride. What does your route pass? And when does that get busy? Riding past schools at the start or end of their day can be very exciting for the practical cyclist. That's why I try to avoid them. Some businesses get busy during rush hour or lunch time (gas stations, fast food outlets, bakeries) — and are also best avoided. Large shopping centers can be busy any time of day, but are worse as they open and close. Unless you are headed to these places, they are best avoided by taking roads that don't go near them. Go around. It will make for a happier ride.

Another map that's good to have is a traffic count map. Not every area has one, but if they do, you want one. (Again, try your local government planning agency.) Traffic count maps show you the average daily traffic count at a given point on a specific road: how many cars go past that spot every day. While these maps don't usually show the counts for minor residential back streets, they will, when you have to take busier roads, help you choose the road somewhat less busy. Not a bad choice.

All right then, you've got your maps, you've got your route, you're ready to go!

But What If It's Dark Out?

When it comes to night riding, there are two basic schools of thought: the Circus Approach and the Stealth Approach. Let's take the last one first, as it doesn't take much to describe. The Stealth Approach is what too many bicycle riders do at night: they wear dark clothes and have no lights. They are invisible out there, and only tend to show up as a noisy bump as they bounce off the car's fender. Needless to say, this is not your best approach. Don't be a stealth biker. There's no future in it.

I prefer the Circus Approach. I wear bright clothes, a reflective vest, and have plenty of lights and reflectors on my bike and person. I am, at night, Chippie the Electric Bozo. This keeps me safe in at least two ways: first off, everyone sees me. No excuses. I *am* visible. And second, no one wants to hit the crazy person on the bicycle. So I get the pity vote, too. Hey, it works for me. Or has so far. Rolling Disco Inferno — that's the look you want to go for. Or at least wear a white shirt.

There is something sublime about riding out under the full moon. Must be the werewolf in me. Still, when you ride at night you need to know that you are not all that easy to see, even with all the lights and reflectors. Drivers do not expect to see a cyclist at night. (OK, few expect to see you in the middle of the day either.) It's also very difficult for a driver to judge the speed of a cyclist any time, and they invariably think you are going much slower than you are. (Quick little thing, aren't you?) The best advice I've ever read on the subject applies to any time of day: treat every driver like they don't see you and the ones that see you like they don't care. Words to live by. Whatever you do, don't *not* ride at night — it is a truly wonderful experience. (Insert werewolf howl here.)

But What If It's Raining?

Yes, it's going to rain. You can count on it. And yes, you will, at some point, be miles from home facing dark clouds. Such is the life of the practical cyclist. It's not that bad. I hate to get wet — just ask my wife. I really do dislike it, and I don't know why. Nevertheless, I honestly don't mind riding my bicycle in the rain. It is somehow therapeutic. It also smells better. Maybe that's what I like about it — the smell of the rain.

There are, however, some things you have to consider when you ride in the rain. A rain storm, unless you live along the Equator, will probably make it cooler. You need to be ready for that. Unless you have a coaster brake or enclosed hub brake, your stopping distances are about to get longer. You need to be ready for that, too. Nothing like hitting the brakes and watching in horror as nothing at all happens. I once tried to get in out of a tropical downpour by riding into an open vegetable market. I hit my hand brakes, nothing happened, and I went right through the market and out the other side. It was all very amusing for all concerned. Even me — eventually. Plan on having seriously reduced brakes. Ride accordingly. (Slower!)

And of course, visibility in the rain is reduced over what we all can see on a bright, bright, sunny-shiny day. (So much for seeing clearly *now*.) The thing to understand here is that not only can you, the bicycle rider, not see as clearly, neither can any of the motorists around you. As a matter of fact, they have a worse view, as they have to look through the rain-streaked windshield. Make sure you always give drivers the benefit of the doubt in the rain. They probably don't see you at all. Give them plenty of room. Then give them some more.

When I ride in the rain, I usually use at least one headlight and one tail light, just so I show up. I usually don't use all of my lights, because I don't want to get them all wet. One of each, front and back, is not a bad idea.

The big deal about rain is that you're going to get wet. I know that's seriously stating the obvious, but you have to know the truth: it's almost impossible to stay dry in the rain. I know. I've tried. You've got several options here when it comes to you, rain, and "dry." The easiest thing to do is to simply go ahead and get wet. It's the cheapest option, and takes the least effort. You don't have to haul anything. Just promise me you will wipe the bike down when you get home. (You'll probably have to do that anyway, no matter what you do to stay dry.)

For some years, I used a two-piece yellow plastic rain suit and overboots to combat the rain. They worked OK: the pants came way up, almost to my armpits under the long jacket, and the overboots kept my shoes dry for the most part. It all worked, but it took three forevers to put on — and if I got caught out in the rain, with no place to hide, I'd be wet by the time I was dressed for it. Also, it did nothing to keep the bike dry. There had to be a better way. And there was.

These days, I use a cycling-specific rain cape. (For a while, I wore the rain suit pants under the cape, but that was just too cumbersome and didn't really add that much to it.) The bicyclist's rain cape has no side openings like a regular (cheap) plastic poncho, and it has loops in the front to hook over either your thumbs or the hand brake levers. It also has a strap that goes around your waist from the back to keep the back of the cape down as you ride. It's cut long enough to go over your handlebars in the front and to cover you completely in the back to keep you dry. It works well: it is bright yellow with a piece of reflective material in the back to help make you more visible in traffic. Mine is made of a treated (coated) woven synthetic material (nylon?) and is light enough to be worn in my warm climate. It also is held out there away from my body, allowing air to circulate beneath it, so I don't get all drenched in sweat when I wear it in the rain. That's good, too. I have had to re-waterproof it at least once, and I've sprinkled corn starch on the inside of it to keep it from sticking together, as it lives most of its long life bundled up in the bottom of my backpack. But it does work, and it works well. For riding in the rain, the cyclist's rain cape gets the Uncle Chippie Thumbs-Up.

You might also get by with simply holding up an umbrella as you ride, but that would only work in a light rain, with virtually no wind. Not the sort of rains we get around here. Some of ours have their own names. I try to not ride in those.

The most serious concern when it comes to riding in the rain is not the rain. It's the lightning. I live where lightning is a grave concern throughout the summer months, and we do get some spectacular lightning storms. Truly frightening. Please take lightning seriously. If you can hear the thunder, it's too close. No need to count the seconds to figure how far away it might be (five seconds to the mile, by the way), just get inside. Now. Please. Deep-fried cyclist is not a happy treat.

Ever seen blue sky lightning? I have. It's amazing, and exactly what it sounds like: lightning out of a clear blue sky. Needless to say, when you see blue sky lightning, it's time to go inside. *Right now.* I do much prefer to see the green flash.

Rain's not so bad — we can deal with rain. Take lightning seriously, and seek shelter if you're at all worried about the weather. There's a big, thick, heavy line between fun and dangerous. This is supposed to be fun. Let's keep it that way.

But What If It's Cold?

OK, look, maybe I'm not the very best person to ask about riding in the cold. I live (on purpose) where it's warm. If I ride once a year when the temperature is near freezing, that's more than enough for me. Still, I do live near sea level, where we also have to contend with thick air and humidity, so "cold" here happens at a much higher temperature. For me, here, staying warm all comes down to layering, air pockets, and windproofing. Oh, and no wool. I don't do wool.

Layering is the classic response to cold, and works well here, where we're all peeling off layers like an old onion by noon. The thing is, you need to vary your layers. Start with tightly woven, thin (comfy!) layers close to the skin, but add bulky, air-trapping layers out from that. Lightweight insulated vests and coats work very well in the cold because they trap air your body can easily warm — but only if you can keep that trapped air warm. The key to that is windproofing the outer layer. Make sure you top it all off with a good windproof jacket — preferable one that's brightly colored.

A perfect cold-weather layering for me would be something like this: a cotton long-sleeve t-shirt under a long-sleeve cotton flannel shirt under a fleece vest under a bulky cotton sweater under a nylon (synthetic) windproof jacket. That will get me through just about anything here, but here is probably warmer than there. And after living here for as long as I have, I do get cold easily. So there.

An Uncle Chippie Hot/Cold Weather Tip: safety glasses. When it gets cold, I wear a pair of clear safety glasses when I ride. It keeps the wind off my eyeballs, and that feels *much* better. I also wear a "turtle fur" neck wrap and wear my heavy leather motorcycle gloves, but that's just me. I get cold just writing about it.

But What If It's Hot?

Ah, now we're talking! I live at a latitude just south of New Delhi, India — but nowhere near New Delhi, India. That means I can ride my bicycle in relative comfort all year around, even through the heat of summer. The key to riding in the heat is comfort, and that means lightweight, light-colored, loose-fitting clothes. I do much prefer cotton, as it breathes well in our humidity. By far the coolest thing I have found to wear on a hot day is a long-sleeve white cotton shirt. Yes, *long-sleeve*. Those long white sleeves will keep your arms cooler than if they were left exposed to the hot, bright sun. The trick here is to wear clothes that allow air to circulate around you, through breathable fabric, but still shade you from the sun. And white — stark, bleached white — is the shade preferred. It really does make a difference.

The other way to keep cool when you ride in the heat is to ride in the shade. I know you can't *always* ride in the shade, but you can, to some degree, choose to ride on tree-lined streets and stay on the shady side of those. Seek the shade of buildings and trees and that will help you keep your cool. Summer is a great time for a ride in the park, under all of those trees!

Also, don't forget: you need to drink a lot more fluids when it's hot and you're out riding. I try to mix sport drinks and water, to end up with a sort of 50/50 balance of the two. You can mix them in one bottle or simply alternate, drinking one and then the other, but do drink liquids when you ride in the heat. Sport drinks offer the ability to replace electrolytes your body uses in the heat, so they are good to have, but you need not drink them exclusively. Drink before you're thirsty — and drink more after that! I go through a lot of liquids here in the summer, but I do keep my cool.

I enjoy riding in the heat of summer where I live, but it does take some getting used to. I ride more slowly, and try to plan my rides for early mornings or in the evenings — out of the heat of the day. With a little planning, the heat shouldn't stop you. Sweat is good, right?

But What If It's Windy?

Ah, the wind — the hill that never ends. Or so they say. The biggest mistake I make in the wind — and I do this all the time — is that I don't check the wind direction before I set off on a bike ride. I just go and ride whichever way I want to ride, only to find that I've been riding downwind for hours (and making very good time) — and now have to ride all the way back, right into it! The moral of the story here is: check the wind direction *before* you leave! I know you can't always ride upwind first. Sometimes you have to go where you have to go, but if you have any choice in the matter at all, ride into the wind first. You will be very glad you did later. Trust your Uncle Chippie on that one.

About the only other thing you can do for a long into-the-wind ride is to gear down — if you have a multi-speed bike — and simply churn away in that easier, lower gear. Tell yourself you're building character. Lie to yourself. That's what I do. Promise yourself great rewards if only you make it back through the wind. That works, too.

The one other thing you can do is to seek wind shadows. Trees, buildings and lower elevations are all great for blocking the wind, at least for part of your ride. Of course, if it's hot out, the wind will help keep you cool and might not be such a bad thing. Then again, if it's cold out, it's the last thing you need. Plan accordingly.

But What About The Hills?

Although I live where it's mostly flatish, we do have hills here and high bridges. I don't mind the hills where I live, but you would probably look at them and laugh. These are hills? Yes, they are if you live here. Hills will humble you. Even small hills. Depending on the bike I'm riding and the hill I'm facing, I take one of two possible approaches to hills. OK, three, counting walking.

If the hill is short and I'm on a single-speed bike (and I have no choice in the matter), I attack. I get up off the seat and really push up the hill. I usually find myself going faster at the top of the hill than I was at the bottom. This works very well with a fixed-gear bike, by the way, as mine seems to *love* hills. No idea why.

If the hill is longer and I am on a multi-speed bike, I let the bike go through a series of downshifts as I climb the hill, almost always ending up in the lowest gear. From there, it's just a matter of churning the pedals 'round and 'round until I reach the top of the hill. I do promise myself I will stop at the top and admire the view. If the hill is, in fact, one of our tall fixed-span bridges, then yes, I will stop. The view is always beautiful.

Don't be afraid to walk the hill. I do it all the time. Get off, push the bike, and save your legs and knees. No shame in that. It can go much worse for you if you force yourself to climb a grade beyond your means and hurt yourself in the process. No glory there. There's no virtue in pain. Not really. Hills can be great training exercises, but you have to approach them, quite literally, with some sense of reason and an understanding and appreciation of your ability at that moment. In climbing there is glory — if you make it.

The flip side of the uphill is, big shock here, the *down*hill. This is what you just did all of that work for. This is what makes the sweat worthwhile: the blast of air and rush of speed as you careen down the far side of the hill, tears streaming from your eyes and dogs giving up the chase as you pass cars left and right. Or maybe not. As thrilling as they are, downhills have their own hazards. The first, of course, is speed.

Few people understand or appreciate how fast a bicycle can go on level ground. Tell them how fast you've gone downhill, and they will think you a liar. They have no idea. I do. We can go *fast.* Be very careful flying downhill, as cars will invariably pull out in front of you. They will do it every time. They have no idea how fast you are going.

Turns going downhill can be real challenges as you'll have to lean your bike over much further than normal to get around the bend. This means you might want to slow down for the turns, and that means you need to use your brakes on the straightaway — and not so much in the turn itself. It's too easy to overbrake in a tight, high-speed turn and slide out, so do most of your braking before the turn. You also want to keep your inside pedal up in the turn. No need to drag a pedal through the turn, and end up with a close, personal relationship with the plant life alongside the road. Inside pedal up. Every time.

Also, don't ride the brakes. I know you might get going fast, but if you ride the brakes too much, that overheats the rims, which overheats the air in the tires — which can expand and blow the tire off the rim. That lives in the house that Jack built. Whew. Go easy on the brakes, if you can. If you can't, and the hill is really that steep and long, do have the good sense to pull over and let the rims cool down before continuing. Your tires will thank you if your heirs do not.

And the last (big) consideration of downhills: what's at the bottom? If you don't know — *go slow*. There could be anything down there. Assume that you will have to stop, and don't let the bike go so fast that you can't stop if something shows up in the next split second and you have to stop within your limited line of sight. It can happen. It happens all the time. Don't let it happen to you. If you *can* see to the next horizon, let 'er rip. If not, then you don't know what you don't know — so take it slow. There will always be another — better — downhill.

But What About Dogs?

Hey, I like dogs. I really do. Love 'em. Had one for years. Still, it can be quite frightening to have one come racing out at you, all snarling white teeth and claws. Thankfully, that doesn't happen every often. We have strong leash laws and a coyote problem. Very few loose dogs around here. I do, however, meet a certain loose little Corgi every once in a while on my way to work in the morning, and we race — I mean really race — flat out. It's wild. The thing is, I know the Corgi is only trying to herd me. He wants me back in the pack. If I stop — which I have done — he keeps his distance, gives up, and goes home. The fun's over. Mostly, though, we race, and I shout encouragement to him as we do. What a fun little dog! May all loose dogs be so much fun.

They are not all fun. I know that. You know that some dogs mean business, and you need to know your options when faced with one. One option you do *not* have is outrunning the dog. Unless the dog is very small, he (or yes, she) is faster than you. Much faster. Your sprint is not that good. Neither is mine. All you can do is talk to the dog, using one of two topics of conversation. Your choice here:

The first approach is my wife's favorite: the "good doggie" tactic. You talk to this full-grown snarling hound as if it were the cutest puppy you ever saw. You confuse the snot out of him. It's a very brave approach and takes serious guts to pull it off — but it works. Yes, you look like a complete idiot baby-talking a carnivorous beast that's about to eat you, but it does tend to calm the dog down. At least enough for you to get out of its territory — and that's the whole point. You are on his turf. Keep moving, no matter what the topic of conversation. The baby talk works — as long as you show no fear. Good luck with that.

The second approach is the "stern father" thing. You tell the dog, in a stern, loud voice, "NO!" and "Go home!" Maybe even point back in the direction the dog came from, on the off chance that might mean something to this animal. You never know. It might. I tend to pick my tactic depending on the apparent seriousness of the dog. If a dog has all the hair up on the back of its neck, it gets the stern father thing. If not, I go for cute doggie. One of the two usually works.

So does stopping, getting off the bike, and walking out of range. Dogs seem to naturally get all excited about anyone on a bicycle. Maybe it's the speed, I don't know, but I do know that some dogs just don't like to see people on bikes. Get off the bike and walk, and now you're OK. Now you look normal, and dog will usually relax somewhat. Still, do *not* take your eyes off the dog. And this is very important: if you do get off the bike, get off on the side *away* from the dog. *Always* keep your bike between you and the dog. It is your last line of defense. Use it.

What not to do? Easy: don't try to hit the dog. Not with your tire pump, not with a stick, not with anything. You are not that fast, nor are you that coordinated. A friend of mine once took a swipe at a dog with his long frame pump as he rode, and proceeded to put said long pump into his front wheel. Hilarity ensued, as did a spectacular end-over-end accident. The dog died laughing. Don't even pretend you're going to hit the dog. They take serious offense at that, and will respond accordingly. And they don't bluff.

By the way, do not be put off by any dog's size, or the lack thereof. A small dog can be just as dangerous as a big dog — maybe more so. Small dogs know no fear and tend to get all carried away when they attack. They can misjudge their speed and yours and end up in your wheels. It's all fun and games until you have to spend the afternoon cleaning the dog out of your bike with a garden hose. Nobody wants that.

If it comes down to it, and you have no choice, yes, a personal defense pepper spray or dog repellent spray will work. It *will* stop the dog. Any dog. I know that for a fact. I know it will work on very large, very serious dogs that mean you much harm. It is, in the words of a friend in law enforcement, respect in a can. Use it wisely if you have to. These days, I don't even carry it at all. I so seldom have a problem with any local dogs, it's hardly worth the effort.

Maybe I owe the coyotes.

A Word Or Two About Car Doors

My friend Michael asked that I mention car doors, so here you go, Michael: car doors. There. Happy? Seriously, what Michael meant was that you have to be careful about not riding so close to parked cars that if someone opens their door, you run into it. While this sounds more like a big-city problem (and Michael does live in a big city), you have to know that it can happen anywhere, anytime. So give any parked car (even a seemingly empty one) a better-than-door-wide berth. You'll be glad you did, and so will Michael. (Thank you, Michael.)

BASIC BICYCLE REPAIR
(Very Basic)

THE FIRST SENTENCE IN THIS BOOK — THE VERY FIRST THING I TOLD you — was that this book is not meant to be a bicycle repair manual. And I want very much to keep that promise to you — it's just that there are a few things you'll need to know to keep your bike in good running order. There are things you'll need to know about your bike to make sure you get home when you go out. Small things, but important things. Mostly, you need to know about tire things.

Of all the things that can go wrong with your bike, the one thing that can stop you in your tracks is a flat tire. Yes, it is technically possible that you could break a drive chain, but I have to tell you: I have never seen that happen. Not on my bikes, and not on anyone else's. I don't recall even hearing of it happening. So let's not worry about that. Let's worry about tires. You can break a cable (either gear or brake) and still get home, only slightly inconvenienced. The seat can fall off and you can pedal standing up. Yes, if a pedal falls off it's awkward — but when does that ever happen? Never. It's all about the tires. Let's talk about your bicycle's tires.

All About Bicycle Tires (And Tubes)

The very best thing you can do for you and your bicycle is to keep your bicycle's tires pumped up to the recommended pressure imprinted on the side of the tire. That will help keep the tire from picking up debris that may puncture the tube, and it will make every ride that much easier for you with noticeably less effort. When I say, "Keep your bike tires pumped," I mean it.

All tires and tubes leak air. Bicycle tires, car tires, truck tires, airplane tires, you name it — if it has an air-filled tire on it, that tire is constantly seeping air. And as long as you know that, it's OK. You can deal with it. High-pressure bicycle tires need to be topped off at least once a week. More casual low-pressure tires should be checked and filled at least once every two weeks. I know of no air-filled bicycle tire that can go a month without being seriously low on air. It's just the nature of the beast. Check your tires once a week.

Yes, low tires give a more comfortable ride. They're squishy soft. It's like riding on water balloons. But that also makes the ride wobbly, you have to pedal harder, and you're far more likely to get a "pinch flat" if you hit something and compress the tire and tube between the ground (whatever you just hit) and the rim. Pinch flats, often called "snake bites," look just like that: two holes, side by side, where either side of the rim bit the tube as it got smashed. Congratulations: now you have *two* holes to patch! Keeping your tires pumped prevents that. And it makes a huge difference in the feel of the bike and the ease of the ride.

You might also consider "thorn resistant" tubes. These are tubes that are much thicker than normal ones, especially on the side they present towards the outside of the tire — toward the ground. Yes, they do help, but there's no such thing as "thorn proof." Thorns stay up late at night, thinking up new ways to make your bike tires go flat. I'm convinced that they do. They must.

There are a couple of downsides to those thicker tubes. They are harder to install. Sometimes *much* harder. Conversely, they can be harder to remove when you do need to repair them — and you will — and harder to work on because of their inherent thickness.

You will also feel the additional weight of that heavier tube as you pedal. Revolving weight on a bicycle's wheels is much more noticeable than static weight on the frame. If you don't mind the heavier pedaling effort, thicker thorn resistant tubes might keep your tires rolling a bit longer. No guarantees.

You can also keep your thinner tubes and add tire liners to help prevent flats. These are heavy, harder strips of plastic that go between the tube and the tire, theoretically preventing anything that got through the tire from touching the tube. That's the theory. In practice, anything that went through the tire should have no trouble going through the tire liner, as it is actually thinner than the tire itself. Just a little bit of logic there.

Also, tire liners can be difficult to install and tend to slide around as you try to fit them in, install the tube, and remount the tire on the rim — so, well, you never do know quite where they end up.

One of the easiest things to do is squirt a bunch of tire sealant into your tubes. I used to do this all the time. The sealant is supposed to seal the tube from those long-term slow seepage leaks as well as plug any small hole you might get. That's what it's *supposed* to do. In reality, what it does is add a weird sloshing weight to each wheel and make it impossible to patch the tube when you *do* get a flat. And you will. Even with this stuff. I don't use tire sealants any more.

In olden times, when dinosaurs roamed the earth, bicyclists used "flint pickers." These were simply cleverly bent pieces of wire that rode along on the surface of each tire and brushed off anything the tire tread might have picked up *before* it got imbedded in the tire and maybe punctured the tube. I used to see these all the time on the serious cyclists' bikes. You don't see them much any more. Still, it seems like the best idea of the bunch.

I have a very simple approach to flat prevention: I carry a spare tube, a patch kit and a pump. That has gotten me home every time. In reality, I only seem to get about one flat a year — except in years when I get more.

All About Bicycle Tire Pumps — And Why You Might Want One

Let me make this perfectly clear: you cannot blow up a bicycle tube with your mouth. Don't even try. They taste really bad. Consider that fair warning, and please don't ask.

So you're going to need a bicycle pump. They come in all sizes and prices, and it honestly doesn't hurt to have two: one small one to take with you when you ride, and a larger one to keep at home. Don't ask how many I have. I'd have to go count. If you only buy one pump (at least to start with), make it the small "minipump" you can take with you when you ride. You can buy the larger "at home pump" later.

I keep a small, no-brand minipump in the tool kit I carry with me whenever I ride. It works well, and it has, on many occasions, gotten me home. Do make sure that you try any pump before you buy it, to ensure you're comfortable with it, know how to use it — and know that it works. I've bought more than one pump that just did not work for me, no way, no how. Test it before you have to.

You can also get longer frame pumps that fasten to the bicycle frame itself. These usually work much better than the minipump I carry, but also require special fittings on the frame to carry said pump. If you have more than one bike, then you would want those same pump fittings on every bike. I carry a minipump in a belt pack no matter what bike I ride. No fittings required. Problem solved. The longer frame pumps do work better, though. Food for thought there.

If you want to go high-tech, you can get pumps that use CO2 cartridges, where you don't have to "pump" at all. I used one years ago, and it worked great, but what do you do if you run out of cartridges? I guess you walk. And carry the bike. The downside is you have to carry a bunch of steel CO_2 cartridges, but the upside is that when you do use the CO_2 pump, the outside of it gets really frosty cold, and that can be kind of nice when you're stuck on the side of the road with a flat on a hot day.

For home use, you can think bigger. Bigger is easier, and easier is good when it comes to pumping up bicycle tires. I have a couple of floor pumps — one at home and one at the office. They work well, move a lot of air, and give me the pressure I need for high pressure tires when I ride them. (I don't always.) Floor pumps are usually designed with a tall, vertical cylinder, topped by a T handle that lets you pump the piston inside the cylinder up and down to inflate the tire on the bike. Most have a couple of little footpads at the bottom that let you literally stand on the pump to steady it as you pump. These are good pumps to have at home, and work great. You should have one.

One pump to avoid is the foot pump. That's an air pump that you work with your foot. I know it sounds like a good idea, but trust me, they don't work all that well. They are awkward to use and tend to flop over as you pump. Very annoying. Avoid. (Personal opinion there.)

I'll tell you the truth: I have a big electric air compressor at home in my garage. It cost as much as a bicycle. It's wonderful. You probably don't need one, but I use mine all the time. I had to learn very quickly that a large air compressor can *really* compress the air. That makes it very easy to blow a bicycle tube into noisy little pieces in about a second if you aren't paying attention. Or even if you are. And while you might not have a big air compressor at home, it is very tempting to use the big air compressor at the local gas station to fill your bicycle tires. You can do it, but it's easy to pop a tube instead. Be careful, and put in much less air than you think you need. Of course, how do you know how much air you put in? You need a tire pressure gauge. A good one.

I have a tire pressure gauge that goes to 150 psi that I keep with my bicycle tools in the garage. I don't carry it with me on the road, but I do use it all the time in the garage. On the road, I just go by feel. I pump the tire until it's about as hard as I think it should be — usually about as hard as I can get it — and hope that's enough to get me home. It usually is. You might want to add a good tire pressure gauge to your list of fun things to buy for your new hobby. It will come in handy. Use it often.

How To Fix A Flat — It's Not That Bad

All right, this is it. You went out for a ride, you're a long walk from home, and that tire is not just soft — it's *flat*. You can't ride on that. Please don't. That just makes it worse. You're going to have to fix it. Right here. Right now. Here's how:

With the bike still right side up, use the brake's cable release (if it has one) to move the brake pads further from the rim to help get the wheel out. If it doesn't have a cable release, don't worry: the flat tire should come right out anyway. (You may have to squeeze it to get it past the brake pads, though.) If the rear tire is flat, and you have any sort of multi-geared bike (internal hub or rear derailleur), put the bike in the highest possible gear. This will let the gear cable go slack and put the chain on a derailleur bike's rear cluster of cogs all the way over to the far right, making it easier to get the wheel off and back on. With an internally geared bike, you have to remove the gear cable from the hub. (You read the instructions that came with the bike, right?) Usually, all you have to do is unscrew the piece where the cable meets the gear-changing mechanism. You don't have to do that with a derailleur bike. Lucky you. Now turn the bike upside down, letting it rest on its seat and handle-bars. Try to avoid ant hills.

If your bike has quick release hubs, turn the quick release lever 180 degrees to loosen the hub from the frame or front fork. Now the front wheel should come right out. With the rear hub, you'll have to work the wheel out, getting the rear cog(s) past the chain, leaving the chain draped on the bike. Once the flatted wheel is off the bike, it's time to get down and get comfy. Find a spot in the shade. Again, try to avoid ant hills.

Remove the small, easily lost cap from the tire's valve. Put it someplace safe, so you can find it next week in the wash. Using your hands, work the tire's bead loose from the rim by pushing inward on it all around the rim, on both sides. The "bead" is the slightly thicker edge of the tire that fits down inside the wheel's outer rim. Each tire has two beads, and there are loops of wire imbedded in them to give them their strength and thickness. Once the tire feels loose on the wheel, use those tire irons you brought along to gently pry the tire's bead over the top of the wheel to the outside of the rim. Be careful to not pinch the tube as you do this, as you can easily cause more problems than you already have. This might be tough at first, getting the tire's bead to the outside of the rim, but it gets easier as you go around the wheel. Once you get the first bead off part way around, it should come loose the rest of the way by you just pulling it out with your hands. Stand the wheel up on end, valve stem at the bottom, and you should be able to remove the other bead from the rim by simply picking it up at the top of the wheel and pulling it off to one side. If not, that's why you still have tire irons. Use them wisely. Mind the tube. Now you have the tire and tube in one hand and the wheel in the other. Or, quite possibly, the tire, tube and wheel in the bushes and a cell phone in one hand. It could go either way.

Assuming that first part went well, you have two choices here: you can do as I like to do, and simply install a fresh, new, unpunctured tube and be on your way the same day; or you can try to patch the tube. Let's try the easy way first: pull out and unwrap your new tube. Unscrew the little valve cap, and see if you can lose this one as fast as you did the first. I know I can. Now stretch the tube out in a couple of directions, like a bad gym exercise. Stretching the new tube helps when you go to tuck it inside the tire. It needs to stretch first, otherwise, it tends to be just small enough to be a real pain to work with and won't tuck inside the tire completely as you install it. With the new (stretched) tube around your neck for safekeeping, pack the old tube away someplace safe. Put it with the valve caps, and you'll never have to deal with it again.

With the wheel flat in front of you, put the tire back on the rim half way — just one bead. Now pull the tire away from the valve stem hole area of the rim, and insert the new tube's valve stem in the hole. Carefully tuck the new tube (this is the *new* tube, isn't it?) into the tire around the rim of the wheel. Once it is all tucked in and comfy, start at the valve stem to tuck the second bead of the tire into the rim. After you get about a third of it seated inside the rim, go back and push the valve stem into the tire a little bit, to allow the tire's beads to settle in under the valve stem. Now finish pushing the tire's second bead over the edge of the rim and onto the wheel. You might have to use your tire irons (Where do you suppose *those* are?) to pry the last of the tire onto the rim. It can be tough sometimes. Be gentle. Be very gentle, as this is the fresh, new tube. The only one you have. No need to pinch this tube and rip it a new one.

Once you've got the tire back on the wheel — check to make sure you didn't leave any tire irons inside the tire (big lumpy bump) — you can put the wheel back on the bike. If you don't pump the tire up until the wheel is back on the bike, it will slide between the brake pads much easier. (So don't.) After you've got the wheel fastened securely in place, and the chain and gear cable tight (if it's the rear wheel), you're ready to pump the tire up. Check, as you pump, to make sure the tire looks even on the rim — no high spots or low spots. Low spots are better than high spots. You can live with low spots. Beware of high spots, though: the tire can pull off the rim right there when you inflate it, and the tube could burst. Bad thing there, unless you have more tubes. Pump the tire up using your handy-dandy minipump. Try to get it about as hard as the other tire, which *should* still be good. With the tire pumped, you're ready to put the bike back on its wheels, pack away your tools and forget all about those valve caps until wash day.

Whoa, what's that you say? You *didn't* bring a spare tube? You brought a patch kit instead? Oh, aren't you the brave one!

In truth, I ride with both a spare tube *and* a patch kit. No optimism here. All right, here we go: let's patch that tube!

Obviously, much of what I wrote above still applies. Once you get the wheel off the bike and the tube out of the tire, instead of packing the old tube away, you're going to want to sit down (away from the ants) and inflate that flat tube with your minipump. This allows you to feel around the tube to find the hole where the air is escaping. If you can't feel it with your hands, try holding the tube close to your far more sensitive eyes — they will feel the cool rush of air. Once you find the hole (and hopefully it's just one — and a small one), either mark it with a pen (that I'm sure you brought) or keep your thumb on it. It's truly amusing to carefully place a tube patch right *next* to the hole. I love it when that happens. I laugh for seconds on end. Maybe three. Now deflate the tube again without losing track of the hole you have to patch. No, I'm not joking. You'll need to push down on the little metal stem inside the valve. Another reason to carry a pen.

Using the little piece of sandpaper in your patch kit, scuff up the tube all over and around the hole (an area slightly larger than the patch you plan to use). Now spread a layer of glue over that area from the insanely small tube of glue that came with your patch kit. Let that glue dry. For me, that's the toughest part: waiting for the glue to dry. Once the glue is dry — and not before — peel the backing off of a patch and set it carefully (but firmly) over the hole. Press it in place with your hands. That's it. You're done. You did it — assuming you did.

Now before you put that tube back in the tire as I described above, feel around the inside of the tire with your bare, ever-so-sensitive fingers, to see if there still might be something stuck in the tire that made the tube go flat. If so, pull it out! No need to go through all of that again! Once you've checked for problems, remount the tube and tire on the rim, reinstall the wheel on the bike, make sure it's tight, pump it up, and Chip's your uncle. You did it!

Bon voyage!

Chains — And Why They Matter

I take a minimalist's approach to chains. The less I have to do with them, the better. I keep mine clean and dry and lightly lubed. Just enough lube to keep the chain from rusting. Any more than that, and the excess lube tends to gather dirt and sand, and that is not good for the chain. Use the least amount of chain lube possible, and keep your chain clean and dry. That works for me (and my chains), and has for years.

I was not going to tell you much more about bike maintenance, since I keep saying that this is not a bicycle repair book, but my friend and longtime bike shop owner Dick Phillips insisted that I tell you how to put the chain back on your bike when it falls off. He said this was the most common problem he had run across in his years in the bicycle business, and it deserved a mention in my book. OK, yes, I've seen it happen, so here goes:

Some time ago I was riding down a bike trail and came upon a woman pushing a brand-new bike. I asked if she was all right, and she said no, she was most decidedly not. The bike had stopped working, and she had no idea why. She was not the least bit amused by this, as it really was a brand-new bike.

I looked down and saw that the chain had fallen off the front chain rings and was between the rings and the seat tube. (Dick was right!) I told her to stop walking for a moment, laid my bike down, reached over, and fixed it in less time than it took for me to type this. She was suitably impressed. (As well she should have been.) (OK, not really.)

If you have a bike with a front derailleur, it's easy for the derailleur to sort of "overderail" the chain. More often than not, that means it will dump the chain onto the frame between the seat tube and your smallest chain ring. In a more spectacular variation on this theme, it might also dump the chain to the outside of your largest chain ring — and onto your right foot. Hilarity ensues, as you might imagine. Even single-cog bikes are not immune to chain drop, but all are easily fixed.

For derailleur-equipped bikes such as the one I encountered that day, all you have to do is grab the chain in front of the bottom of the rear derailleur, and pull it forward and up over the front chain ring(s), placing it on the ring that most closely matches the position of the front derailleur. That will be the easiest one to put it on anyway. That's it. You're done. It was that easy.

If the chain has come off both the front chain ring and the rear cog (this is more common on single-cog bikes), turn the bike upside down and put the chain over the front chain ring first. Now you can turn the pedals as you carefully direct the moving chain over the rear cog. Watch your fingers. In this case, the chain came off because it was too loose. You can be a real hero if you loosen the rear wheel and pull it back a bit, tightening the chain. You are now, officially, a bicycle hero.

Go team.

Everything Else ... That Matters

This is not a bicycle repair book. This is not a bicycle repair book. This is not ... OK, yes, there are still some things you need to know about maintaining your bike. Little things that will make sure it works well and lasts a long time. These aren't things that will stop you dead in your tracks, but knowing how to deal with them will make your bike rides that much better. Like I said, the little things.

If you have hand brakes, then you have brake pads, and those pads do call for attention from time to time. They wear out, pick up debris, and sometimes squeal. You can tell a brake pad is worn out if you can't see the grooves that were original- ly cut in the braking surface of the pad. (Sort of like tread on a tire.) When the treads on your brake pads are gone, its time for new pads. Just like tires.

If the brakes make a nasty grinding sound when you use them, it's time to pull them off and clean them. This usually takes a small metric wrench or metric Allen wrench, but is not an impossible task. Clean the surface of the brake pad with sandpaper, a metal file or, if you're me, about one wild second on a grinding wheel. I don't mess around.

If your brakes squeal, that often means they need more "toe in," that is, the leading edge of the brake pad needs to hit the rim first. If it does not, the pad's position can often be adjusted to make that happen. Failing that, you'll have to sand the pad down to create that angle. Is the squeal really that bad?

Cables, both gear and brake, do rust and wear out. Mostly, they rust. When they get sticky rusty, it's time for new cables. A little grease on the cables does help. I grease them before I install them, but pulling them out just to grease them isn't all that much fun. This is a bike shop thing, as some gear cables are virtually impossible to replace — you have to replace the entire gear shifting mechanism. (I am *not* a big fan of those systems.)

It is also possible to break a gear or brake cable, although it does take considerable effort. If you start to see loose little wires coming undone from the cable, usually at one end or the other, it's breaking slowly. If it's breaking slowly, replace it fast. And by the way, if you need to replace one cable on your bike, it's not a bad idea to replace all of them at the same time. They are all about the same age, are they not?

Pedals lead a hard life, right down there near the street and almost always in the dirt and puddles and debris. They do wear out, and they do break. (The inexpensive plastic pedals that come on so many bikes today wear out and break just that much faster.) Thankfully, they are not that hard to replace. You can do it at home with a 15mm open-end wrench. Just remember that the left side pedal always threads on (and off) backwards. Righty-tighty, lefty-loosey becomes, um, lefty-tighty, righty-loosey. Don't say you weren't warned. Put a little dab of grease on the new pedal's threads before you put it on the bike. That will make your life easier later. And buy better pedals than the ones you are replacing. You'll be glad you did.

The quickest way to damage a pedal is to leave the inside pedal down in a turn and scrape it on the ground. This is bad for the pedal, and may pitch you off into the bushes with little warning. Unless you enjoy that sort of thing, it could be bad for you, too. Keep your inside pedal up through the turn. That means don't pedal through the turn. If you're on a fixed-gear bike, and have no option to coast, at least know how far you can lean the bike before you become one with the bush. Be nice to your pedals. They get you home.

Spokes? Ah, spokes! There's nothing quite like the subtle metallic sound of a spoke breaking to take all the love and joy out of a ride. That soft, gentle "PING!" that tells you that you are now, officially, skating on thin ice — and much further from home than you thought. For the most part, breaking one spoke is not the end of the ride. But it is the harbinger of a larger problem with that wheel — usually the rear wheel. (Why is it always the *rear* wheel?) Start breaking more spokes, and you've got a problem.

Not all bicycle wheels use tensioned wire spokes, but yours probably does. A tensioned wire spoke wheel is a thing of great beauty and can be a joy forever — if you're lucky. The trick to it is making sure that all of the spokes in the wheel are evenly tensioned. This is not an everyday fuss around the garage thing. This is an art form. For the average practical cyclist, you may only need to know how to deal with a broken spoke once in a great many years. They do last a long time.

If you have broken a spoke, you may or may not hear it. It sounds like a metal softball bat connecting with a slow-pitched ball: a good, solid "PING!" Once you've heard it, you know the sound — and hate cycling past softball fields in season. A good game can be so distracting. Was that a spoke?

If you discover a broken spoke on your bike, the first thing to do is spin the wheel to make sure it clears the brake pads. If it does, all you can do then is pedal home *gently* and make arrangements to get the bike — or at least the wheel — to the bicycle shop to have them replace the spoke and retrue (and retension) the wheel. Many art forms involved there, and maybe some special tools — a spoke wrench, at the very least.

If the wheel with the broken spoke does hit the brake pads, you might want to loosen the brake's setting, allowing more room between the pads for the now-warped rim, or remove one or both pads entirely so they don't rub on the way home. Ride softly.

More often than not, the loss of one spoke is not a ride ender. If it is, and the wheel is seriously, dangerously warped, all you can do is dismount and walk. Yes, I have replaced spokes on the road, but to do that, you have to carry the right length spare spokes (your bike uses at least two different lengths, and maybe three), a spoke wrench, and a device to remove the rear freewheel or gear cassette if the broken spoke is on the drive side of the rear hub. (And it most often is.) Been there, done that, but not for many years. You shouldn't ever have to worry about this, but if you do, there you go: all about spokes.

Is That All You Need To Know About Bike Repair?

That depends. How much more do you want to know? There are whole, huge, thick books out there on the glorious subject of bicycle repair. There are whole, huge, great schools that teach the subject gloriously. All you need to know right now is enough to make sure you get home if you have a flat, drop a chain, or maybe pop a spoke. Little else goes wrong out on the road. That's not to say it won't, but it usually doesn't. (Famous last words there, I know.)

I can go for long months at a time and never have a thing go wrong on any bike. Just pump up the tires and ride. No flats, no worries. I like that. Then again, my fortunes can change, I can find myself spending long evenings out in the garage patching endless flat tubes and wondering how long that spoke has been so very broken. And why didn't I notice it before? Oh, bother.

For the most part, if you keep your bike clean and dry and keep the tires pumped up, you won't have any problems at all. Just ride your bike and enjoy the ride. As much as I do enjoy working on bikes, they really are more fun to ride than they are to work on.

Concentrate on the riding.

10

WHAT HAPPENS NEXT? ... And What After That?

THERE IS SIMPLY NO WAY I COULD PUT EVERYTHING ABOUT BICYCLES and bicycling in this one little book. There's so much else to it, and yet it's still a wonderfully simple way to get around. For now, this is what you need to know to get started. This is just the beginning.

I recommend that you make friends with everyone at your local bike shop. Get to know them, know what they sell, and know what they can do for you to get you out on the road on the right bike, set up correctly for you. The folks at that bike shop have all been riding for years, but they all started out just like you with a first bike and a first ride.

Don't get discouraged. The riding gets easier. I often set off on a morning on my bike and have to remind myself that the first few minutes don't count. Let yourself ride for a distance, get warmed up, and see a few sights. You'll feel much better and go even further when you give yourself a chance to get into the rhythm of the ride. (And all rides have a rhythm.) Failing that, drop down a gear. You probably aren't spinning like I told you. There you go — isn't that better?

Pick destinations that make you happy. Nothing wrong with a bicycle ride to the ice cream shop! See, you're happy already. You can justify the all-you-can-eat Chinese buffet if you ride the long way around to get there, and the long way home as well. Read a travel book at the library as your bicycle is securely locked up outside, awaiting your next travel and adventure. Better still: bring a book with you when you ride your bicycle to the park, pick a shady tree, and have a good read with your trusty bike right there beside you. Wear your bicycle helmet and cycling gloves in the grocery store and see if anyone asks. They usually will.

As the Practical Cyclist (note the capital letters there), you will meet and greet other cyclists now wherever you go. It's inevitable. It's like a cult. One of the good ones: the Cult of the Bicycle. No secret handshake, though. Not yet, anyway. (I need to work on that.) Bicyclists just naturally gravitate. We have much in common. We share the same roads, the same hills, and the same weather. We're all out there. Do stop for other cyclists that may need your help, even if you have no idea what you're doing. Sometimes they just need to see a smiling face on another bicycle. If nothing else, you can walk together, pushing the bikes. Be the friend on the bike.

Getting Your Bike There Without Riding It There

You know that the bicycle is not a stand-alone form of transportation, right? You can always mix and match it with other ways to get around. More often than not that means putting your bicycle in — or on — your car and driving somewhere to ride your bike. I know that sounds counter-productive, but sometimes that's a great way to ride someplace that would be difficult to ride *to*.

If your bike is small enough and your car is big enough, you can put your bike in your car and off you go. Sometimes that means you have to remove the front wheel (easy enough to do), and it always helps to have a heavy blanket to protect the interior of your car from your bike, but that is the very best way to get your bike somewhere else, keeping it safely locked in your car as you go. (Safer to stop for lunch.)

With smaller cars and bigger bikes, a bicycle rack is the way to go. The big choice here is between a mount on the roof and a mount on the bumper. I like the racks that mount on the bumper, if only because I don't have to think about it before I come home and drive into the low-hanging garage with the bicycles firmly affixed to the roof. I can't begin to tell you how amusing that's *not*. Bumper-mounted bike racks are the way to go — much easier to load and unload, too. Just make sure you lock your bikes to the rack and/or the car if you plan to leave them unattended enroute.

Locally, the public buses around here all have bicycle racks on the front. Yes, *every* bus. There is no extra charge to bring your bike with you on the bus, using these racks. If you ride a small folding bike, you can always fold the bike up and take it with you inside the bus, thus freeing up the front bike rack for a cyclist who doesn't ride a folding bike. (And conversely, if the bike rack is already full, you still get to bring your bike along for the bus ride.) Yet another reason to ride a folding bike. "Bikes on Buses" is a great idea. My hat is off to whoever came up with it.

When it comes to traveling with your bicycle beyond your personal car or the local bus, there's not much I could tell you that might hold true for everyone, everywhere. Long-distance buses, trains and airplanes are all (for the most part) commercial businesses, and each company or government agency can set its own rules, regulations, conditions and fees when it comes to people bringing their bicycles with them for the trip. You really do need to call before you show up, bike in hand. And if you don't like what they tell you when you call, you need to call someone else. Failing that, you go someplace else.

How Do You Know If You're A Practical Cyclist?

So you bought this book, you read this book, and now you ride a bike. Good for you! You rock! But how do you know if you're really a cyclist, practical or otherwise? There are many ways:

- If you've ever walked around the office all morning and not noticed you were still wearing those pant cuff bands from your bike ride in, then yes, you are a real cyclist.

- If someone stops you for directions and you proceed to send them down every twisty little back road in town, there's a good chance that you ride a bike.

- If you talk about hills no one else sees and wind no one else feels, that just means you're the one there on the bike and everyone else drove. That makes you the cyclist.

- If you show up at your destination all wide awake and ready to go, you probably pedaled there, didn't you? Everyone else is in a fog because they came by car. Pity them.

The effects of the bicycle on the human are subtle. You will not notice your legs of steel, but others will. They will speak in hushed tones as you pass. That's OK. You can outrun them if you have to. You will, of course, bore every car driver within earshot with how much fun you are having riding your bike, how much money you are saving, and how great it is to not have to worry about a parking spot whenever you go anywhere by pedal power.

Like any form of exercise, bicycling runs the risk of becoming an addiction, but that's OK. It's a very good addiction. One you can live with. One that will let you live a longer and healthier life. Make the most of both bicycling and your life.

You've Read My Book — Now Ride Your Bike!

If you come away from this little book knowing nothing else, know this: *you can do it*. You can ride a bicycle. You can ride safely, be comfortable, and look good doing it. You can be a practical cyclist. I won't say, "If I can do it, anyone can do it!" but I will say that *almost* anyone can and that certainly more people should.

Ride your bicycle because it's fun. Yes, it makes sense both financially and environmentally, but ride your bike because it's more fun than driving. That, to me, is the best reason of all. If it's not fun, why bother?

Once you try la Vida Velo, you might find it to be quite enjoyable. I know I have. You might (brave prediction here) find it to be better than driving. You will certainly feel better about yourself, and be healthier for the effort. Being a practical cyclist is not a bad thing to be.

Bicycling will also give you a whole different outlook on where you live. You will see places you've never seen before and go down roads you've never ridden. Your neighborhood and your town will both open up as you explore on your bicycle and contract as you become more focused on "Where can I go on my bike?" You will know more about the world around you than you ever knew before. This is going to be fun.

Are there limits to this? Are there limits to how far you can go? Not really. With a little bit of practice and care, you can go anywhere: across town or across the continent, all by bicycle. People do it all the time. Someone is probably doing it right now. A steady pace and a day's effort can put you an amazing distance from home. Here's hoping you get to amaze yourself with how far you've gone on a bicycle.

You want cold, hard numbers? How about these: a person in reasonably good health, on reasonably good roads (and with a decent bike), should be able to cover, with an acceptable level of effort, a hundred miles a day. That's 160 kilometers. Yes, with practice you can do it. It will take all day, eight to ten hours or so, but it is possible. You can, with practice and effort, do it. Can you imagine?

Before you point your bike to the horizon and pedal for all you're worth, just enjoy riding your bicycle in your own neighborhood. That's all you have to do. It doesn't have to be about epic rides or yellow jerseys. No need to stand on the podium and hear your national anthem. Just go for a bike ride to your own place, at your own pace. A trip to the local store, by bike, can be a grand adventure, and all you need to do to feel good about it. The long rides may come in time, but the short rides will always be there for you to enjoy. They will be your favorites.

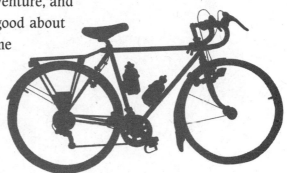

Now go ride your bike.

Index

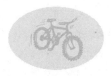

About The Author

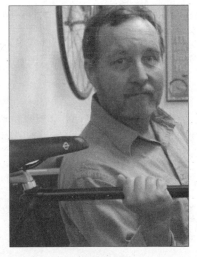

CHIP HAYNES IS A DEVOTED husband, artist, writer, juggler and, yes, practical cyclist living just south of Latitude 28 North with his wife, The Lovely JoAnn, where they own more bicycles than might be reasonably prudent or entirely necessary. Although a graphic artist by profession, Chip has written countless articles on practical cycling for Mason St. Clair's *Wire Donkey* newsletter out of Nashville, Tennessee, USA, and rides his little three-speed folding bike to work every day. (Except on days when he rides one of his other bikes.)

If you have enjoyed *The Practical Cyclist*, you might also enjoy other

BOOKS TO BUILD A NEW SOCIETY

Our books provide positive solutions for people who want to make a difference. We specialize in:

Sustainable Living • Ecological Design and Planning
Natural Building & Appropriate Technology
Environment and Justice • Conscientious Commerce
Progressive Leadership • Resistance and Community • Nonviolence
Educational and Parenting Resources

New Society Publishers

ENVIRONMENTAL BENEFITS STATEMENT

New Society Publishers has chosen to produce this book on recycled paper made with 100% post consumer waste, processed chlorine free, and old growth free.

For every 5,000 books printed, New Society saves the following resources:[1]

20	Trees
1,772	Pounds of Solid Waste
1,949	Gallons of Water
2,543	Kilowatt Hours of Electricity
3,221	Pounds of Greenhouse Gases
14	Pounds of HAPs, VOCs, and AOX Combined
5	Cubic Yards of Landfill Space

---

[1]Environmental benefits are calculated based on research done by the Environmental Defense Fund and other members of the Paper Task Force who study the environmental impacts of the paper industry.

For a full list of NSP's titles, please call 1-800-567-6772 *or check out our web site at:*

www.newsociety.com

NEW SOCIETY PUBLISHERS